Move Over Manic Depression - Here I am!

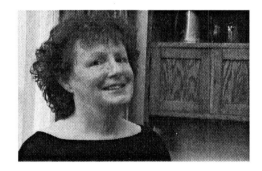

By Anne Brocklesby

"One million people commit suicide every year"
The World Health Organization

Published by:
Chipmukapublishing
PO Box 6872
Brentwood
Essex
CM13 1ZT
United Kingdom

www.chipmunkapublishing.com

This book is dedicated to my mother Ellen O'Hara born 14th August 1915, and who died in July 1972 aged 56 years. She is one of my children's grandmothers.

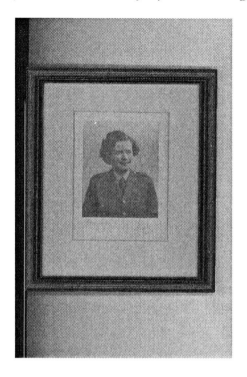

Forward

This book has a caring husband, some people do not even have that. Their love is a good undertone in the book. The family relationship even in life does help heal and care.

Emotions are hard thing to understand at any age and the person feeling alone without being along is understood in this book. At a time when the social skills were different, so were the peer pressures.

This book also addresses issues where you have not had children. Where you have had children you will feel those feelings that you hope not to return.

This is a woman who has had it all and won.

Andrew Latchford
Co Founder

Thank you Andrew. It sometimes has not felt as though I have had it all and won. As time goes on, and I learn insight, and have more understanding of everyone's different positions, then I can feel it is OK. This is life, and I am living it.

Anne Brocklesby, Author, November 2006

Move Over Manic Depression – Here I Am
By Anne Brocklesby

Preface

Chapters

1. An Ordinary Childhood
2. Separation And Anxiety
3. Independent Life At University
4. My Mother's Illness And Death
5. Life Without My Mother
6. Post Natal Depression
7. Miscarriage
8. Difficulties Of Being A Mother Without A Mother
9. My Illness
10. My Husband In His Own Words And How The Family Has Coped With My Illness
11. Marriage And Bringing Up My Two Children
12. The Role Of My Psychiatrist
13. Medication And Self Help
14. Exercise Diet And Lifestyle
15. Anxiety
16. Depression
17. Mania
18. A Diagnosis of Manic Depression
19. Fighting Against The Medical Establishment
20. Alternatives As A Supplement To Traditional Medicine
21. How My Family Coped
22. Poems For Mental Health
23. Psychiatrist's Report

24. Ready To Take A Stand
25. Writing This Book
26. Time To Catch Up
27. The Use of Alcohol As Self Medication
28. The Power Of Prayer
29. Therapy And A Productive Life
30. Remembering My Mother – Some Positive Images
31. Death In The Family
32. Some More Poetry
33. Improving Mental Health In The General Population (paper written September 2001)
34. Post-Script To My Memoirs
35. A Tribute To My Mother-in-Law

Preface

My sister was staying for a few days in September 2003, and we were talking like you do to close family members, and I said, 'I wish I'd never gone to see the psychiatrist'. And my sister said, 'But Annie, you were mad, quite mad'. I mean there was really no choice in the matter; I was taken to see the psychiatrist. And that's the way it was. The weekend I had my real breakdown, I remember well being in floods of tears, and being totally unable to control my feelings. My husband and my sister contacted the GP surgery, as an emergency on the Saturday, and a tranquiliser was prescribed for me with a follow-up appointment on the Monday. My sister moved in to stay over the weekend, and came with us to see the Doctor. A referral was made to the psychiatrist, and I became one of his patients. That was nearly seven years ago now, and over this time I have been on a roller-coaster of emotions, tried various prescribed medicines, and overall just tried to cope with my feelings, and keep some sort of control of my life. I must say that it has been extremely difficult and many, many times I would have given up, but my husband David has been there beside me, always asking questions at the psychiatrist's office when the pills did not seem to be anything like a cure, and he was always ready to cook a meal, to give me a cuddle, to take me for a walk, come to swimming and exercise classes with me, and to let me just relax without the hassle of having to get out and cope with a paid job. Over the years I have tried paid work, and sometimes done voluntary work, but on the whole have not been fit to run an ordinary life at all. It has been a question of just surviving, rather than making any progress. I feel I have been cut off from my previous life style and the friends I would tend to make quite easily. I have become more and more isolated, and with it have lost so much confidence. It is now after seven long years that I am beginning to feel I have got quite a good combination of prescribed drugs and a more defined personal approach to coping with my illness. It is time to say I want to live again, and make time for me. So, I need to say move over and out to the manic depression. You are not going to rule my life as you have been doing, and I am going to cope with life again. This tale is not exaggerated or told for the spin, it is just as it was. The story is not sensationalist, but may in fact be understated. Writing my story is all part of the therapeutic process for me to be able to embrace life again.

This book, as my story, will I hope give others, like yourself or your friend or family member some hope that there is light at the end of the tunnel. Or to put it another way, that although you may be feeling trapped at the bottom of a deep, dark well, there are people at the top looking down trying to find some way of reaching those below. I had been stuck in this well for so long, I had forgotten what it was like to even see the light, let alone think of returning to live in the light. Yet now I feel that there are people there trying to help and so I am not trapped or living in despair. I feel as though I have some energy to put into getting myself better and I can feel some synergy with what is going on around me in the wider world. I want to break free, and these are my words.

Chapter 1- An Ordinary Childhood

I was born the oldest of 3 girls, and have always been close to my sister Joanie, some 3 years younger than myself. I grew up in the 50's, and came to life at 12 with the arrival of the Beatles. I joined their fan club and avidly read absolutely every paper, or magazine or article about them. I lead a quiet family life, going to school, and I was in the Brownies and spent a year in the older group of girls called Guides. My mother took me to dancing classes before I went to school, but the only thing I really remember was the time the teacher responded to my invitation to demonstrate to the class how to do a particular ballet step. When I had proudly finished, the ballet teacher said, now that's how not to do it. I remember to this day, at the age of 52, how I felt absolutely mortified, and sat down shamefacedly. What an encouragement to childhood enthusiasm! At school I did well, because my grandfather, my mother's father, had taught me to read and write before I went to school, so work there was a little boring, and the only way to get some sort of attention from the teacher was to make a deliberate mistake, whereupon the teacher would say to me, 'Now Anne, what's happened to you today?' My father worked five and a half days a week, including Saturday mornings, and my grandfather lived with us until he died when I was 12. I remember my first day at school, being taken by my mother to this new place, where there was a most magnificent tubular steel climbing frame in the tarmac playground. I was scared stiff and knew no one. On my second day I was eating a sweet in the classroom, as I did like sweets at that age, when the teacher told me to take it out of my mouth and put it into the bin!! Thus I learned that you do not eat sweets in school lessons.

On the whole I enjoyed school, and got on OK with my various classmates. I passed the 11+ and I remember being called to the headmistress' office to telephone my mum, and I just said 'I've passed.' So it took my mum a little time to work out what I was talking about, but I was very pleased. I started at secondary school and again I knew no-one, so walked endlessly round the playground at break-times until eventually -it seemed absolutely ages – I made some friends to be with when there were no lessons. It was not too easy for me, because I was rather shy, and so my friendships were limited to a small handful of girls. I remember jealousy reigned supreme. I worked very hard at school work and did well. In those days you just had to get on with making friends the best you could. There was no highly developed social skills learning that girls of today go in for. At the age of 14 we moved from London to Scotland, and my mother became ill with heart trouble. I wanted to change the world, and felt strongly about social injustices and poverty. My parents took the Times and the Telegraph and I wanted to read the Guardian. However, I was a well-behaved, sociable, helpful family member. This continued until I left home at 18 to go to University in Edinburgh to study sociology and the other social sciences.

Chapter 2 – Separation and Anxiety

I think I developed a separation anxiety at a very early age, and had the enduring feeling that in fact I was an orphan. My mother told me that I was sent for 3 weeks to my aunt and uncle's house, with two of their children, to spend time being looked after by them when my mother was giving birth to my sister Kay, her second child. Of course I do not remember any of this, but I am conscious of a feeling of separation, which I can only trace to this time. My mother said that when I returned, I looked like a neglected orphan, because my hair seemed a tangled mass, as though it had not been brushed or combed. Three weeks was a long time to be stationed away from the only security I knew with my mother, to an aunt and uncle who I did not know at all, in a strange house, a journey of some one and a half hours from London. Just see it from my point of view, that on my return, I was presented with a little baby sister, with whom I must have competed for time and attention of _my_ mother. Again, I cannot remember specifically feeling any jealousy towards my sister then, or later, but maybe it was an even deeper feeling that I have never been conscious of. However, throughout my childhood, jealousy towards school-friends always came into the picture. I was the responsible older sister to my two younger sisters, but also liked to laud it over them as the older sister sometimes, when I would chase them around the place, pretending to be a great monster. My middle sister reminded me of some of these games in recent years, which served to bring them to my attention, as I had forgotten those times. On the whole I remembered always being the responsible, older sister, and trying to keep my two sisters in order, as was expected of the older child. However, I also remember visits to the seaside where I was scared to get out of the car to go for a walk onto the beach with my sisters, leaving my parents in the car, and I always had that feeling that they might not be there when I came back. This feeling was a very strong one and I absolutely felt I had to remain in sight of my parents, so that they could not disappear from my view. It was the only way I could keep some sort of control, but of course it did not present like that, and no one could understand why I would not go and play as my two sisters did. But then how could I explain that sort of feeling to my parents at the time? It all tended to come out the wrong way, and I felt stupid, and understood that my behaviour was silly. Yet at the time I did not associate it with my early separation and anxiety.

Later in my teenage years I developed a favourite character in a book. Perhaps I modelled myself on her. My favourite was Maggie Tulliver in 'Mill On The Floss' by George Eliot. Her great need as a young girl was to be loved, and I felt the same, to the extent that I identified with her, feeling that what I needed in my life was to be loved. On one occasion when I had had my nervous breakdown, I remember sitting with my husband in the doctor's surgery, describing my feelings of need like Maggie Tulliver, but making it quite clear, that that was in the past, and now it was OK. So, although these feelings sunk into the back of my consciousness when I read the book at 15, these bare, essential needs of mine were clearly expressed when my emotions were upturned, and I tried to describe how

I was feeling. Of course, this well-known character had a traumatic end when she died trying to save her beloved brother, and they were both swept away together. I can write now, that it was not the tragic end which I had identified with, but perhaps the way in which she had died did make a profound impression upon me. In the same way I can now associate my confirmation saint with the same tragic end. Saint Dorothy, whom I chose at the age of 9 to be my confirmation name, had died as a martyr for her faith, on my birthday, another factor which had drawn her to me. I did tend to be fairly easily influenced by these emotional strings, which pulled me this way and that. At the age of 10 my mother asked me if I wanted to go off to boarding school in Scotland, but I said no, because I was too scared to contemplate living away from my home. I was not even curious enough to ask anything about the prospective boarding school, as I'm sure most children would do.

Chapter 3 – Independent Life at University

This will be a very short chapter indeed, because at university I worked hard. To my shame I am afraid that I did not make many new friends, and I did not join any of the societies, so I did not branch out as it were. However, I was fulfilled doing my academic work and I got good results. I enjoyed the routine of lectures and working in the library, and my independence in the halls of residence. I went to a few parties, and two of the balls. I remember a brief attachment to someone special to me at the time, and I saw him once or twice in London after university finished. I graduated with a BSc (Social Sciences) Magna Cum Laudae which means with distinction and is equivalent to an Upper Second Honours Degree. I left university and Edinburgh at 21, and my middle sister Kathryn, who continued her studies there. My mother died the day after I graduated, in July 1972, and I moved to the London area in the September to start working as a social worker. My mum had been fairly ill throughout my university days, and to some extent I just blanked out all my emotions by working hard, trying to ignore what was going on. I found it all very difficult. Some six weeks or so after my mother's death, my younger sister Joanie, aged 18, and me, aged 21, set off in the car together with all our possessions to start a new life in the south.

At Edinburgh University I studied social sciences, which meant I spent 3 years reading sociology and social administration, my two choice subjects. I found the work very challenging and it totally occupied my attention throughout this difficult part of my life. In addition, there were various other options and I ended up choosing French, Economic History, and Psychology, with Mathematics for Social Sciences, as an additional subject in the third year, just to keep me busy. Occasionally I went home for a weekend to see my mother, but on the whole I preferred to stay in Edinburgh, with the other students. I wish now I had not been so preoccupied at the time with my mother's health, as I could have got myself really involved in university life, like my younger sister Joanie did when she went to Brunel, after our mum had died.

Chapter 4 - My Mother's Illness and Death

To this day, and I'm now 52, I feel great sadness at the illness and death of my mother. She died when I was 21, after a long illness, and frequent hospitalisations. It meant that our family life from my late teens was much curtailed. We did not have great big family outings and experiences because my mother was ill. For example I never remember once being out on a walk with my mother. But I do remember her illness, pain and depression. When she first became ill, when I was 14, the doctor came to the house in the night, and I was terrified she would die. In the morning, my dad told us my mum was unwell, and that she had had a heart attack, and I had that terribly heavy sinking feeling that I still recognise today. She went to hospital for some months, and the house was terribly empty, and I missed my mum. I don't remember ever going to see her. I really can't understand it. Then my mum returned home and we moved to Scotland to live, because my dad had had a promotion at work, and he was relocated. I think my mother had been looking forward to spending time at the London theatres, and enjoying herself now that the 3 children were nearly teenagers, but just at that time came the call to move north. I do not suppose that helped her, but I knew nothing of all this at the time. We moved north and suddenly it was a very different world.

We had been used to Scotland, because we had spent our summer holidays there every year. My parents drove in the car, my grandfather was dropped off to visit his son for two weeks, and we arrived in central

Scotland, to spend our month's holidays. After arriving, our parents would set off for their two weeks without the kids, travelling in Scotland, and as they were both Scottish, I think they enjoyed this part of the holiday, and we three were left with the grandparents. I enjoyed my holidays with my grandmother and her sister, both in their 80's at the time. We were taken around to their various friends, to be shown off, and we had lovely afternoon teas with sandwiches and cakes, and morning coffees sometimes too. Every Friday afternoon we made sandwiches of strawberries, cold meats, and sometimes bananas, and we made tea in the summer house, then waited for the guests to arrive. We always had a tea leaf reading. I did enjoy those times. There was the annual meal in a big hotel with all the relatives, and there were the trips to buy chips, or that special Italian ice-cream. Again, the regular routine of these holidays sticks in my mind. Sometimes we would sit on the dyke in front of the house and take down car numbers, and other times we would play together. We were easily amused. Of course our holidays to Scotland had prepared us for everyday life there, but the change in lifestyle was quite a shock for the family.

I do remember very sad times, when my mother was in hospital over Christmas, and we would go up to the ward, with our presents. I remember my mother asked us one time to give some of the presents to an elderly lady who had no visitors or presents, and so we did. We also spent time talking to her. I'm sure all these experiences made me feel that it was a natural thing to want to help people, and was the reason why I turned initially to social work as a livelihood. I had become a carer. Of course I wanted to change the world, and I wanted the sadness of my life to change too, but that was the way it was. I tried to appear content with the world, but inside I think I was very sore. For me, it was some relief to go off to university at 18 and live away from home, because I did not have the constant reminder of my mother's illness.

I still worried about her, but had the distraction of work. Sometimes she would be in hospital, and I remember most of my university days sending my mother different cards in an effort to keep up the communication and to wish her well. In those days there were no mobile phones, so I phoned when she was at home, and sent cards to her when she was in hospital. She told me the nurses would always be clamouring around her bedside to see what the post had brought in for her that day. My cards became quite famed. Sending cards helped me keep in touch, and it still does to this day, as I will often send a postcard or a greetings card, instead of picking up the phone to say hello.

In my final year in Edinburgh, I think I became quite depressed with the worry over my mother. I think she had been hospitalised most of the time, and both my sisters were now living away from home. One was in Edinburgh, embarking on year two of a 5 year joint honours course, and my sister Joanie had spent the year in Paris as an au-pair, prior to university entrance. I used to worry about my mother and knew that life for her was very difficult. Sometimes I went out on a shopping trip to buy myself something just to cheer me up. After exams in June I went home for the last time, then spent time travelling in Germany before returning for my graduation. My mum entered hospital again when I was away, and never came out. She lost the power of speech too, and took to writing in a notebook. She was in a bad way and I found the last week unendurable. My mum lay in bed dying, and I visited her every day. I did not want to leave her bedside to go to my graduation but my dad encouraged me and came with me, saying my mum would be proud of me. So we went to Edinburgh, and I graduated and got my certificate and the photograph which I hate to this day, because of the awful feelings it arouses. We came back to the hospital after that journey and saw my mother, and that was the last time I saw her alive, because the next morning she was dead. I still find the whole episode quite traumatic, and I have this awful association in my mind of university, graduation and death.

Chapter 5 - Life Without My Mother

My mother was a strong character, and inspired her 3 girls to be equally strong minded individuals. She herself was a university graduate, which was quite unusual in her day. She had held down good jobs before marrying and becoming a mother and housewife which again was the usual route into housewifery. Her father had been a headmaster of a school in Glasgow I believe, and his presence in my early childhood in our family home, had ensured that all three girls could read and write before starting school. I remember we also played tennis with him on the lawn when we were old enough to set up the court and so we had fun with him too. He was a keen gardener, and he encouraged us to grow our own plants from seeds. His wife, my mother's mother had also died of heart trouble at exactly the same age, in mid fifties, as my mother. This has always hung over me, and coloured my thoughts. For example, at 26 I took out my life insurance policy to mature at 55, so that I would get some benefit from it too. At the time I thought that the fifties were a long way off so I did not worry on a day to day basis about my health, but I had the feeling that my life might be cut off at that fairly early age too. However, I have also had the counterbalancing effect of having a grandmother, my father's mother, live to 102, and she was extremely healthy and lived on her own until she was 97, so one can never tell. We are all a mixture of the gene pool and can only influence our health by trying to follow a healthy diet and lifestyle.

I did also search to replace my mother with another mother figure. I once said to my mother-in-law that I treated her as my mother, but she said to me that she could not be my mother. Also, I did become close to my father's second wife, my children's grandmother, but of course she also was not my mother, although she was the second family grandmother. When my stepmother died I had this awful resurgence of grief for my own mother, even though it was some twenty five years after her death. It was as though I had started to get on with my own life after my mother's death, and although I was sad that my mother had died, I also felt enormous relief that she was at peace after all those years of suffering. I also felt relief for myself, that I would no longer have to worry about my mother being ill, and in hospital. So, at the time of my mother's death there was a sense of relief. After my step-mother's death however, it was as though the old wounds had re-opened, and I felt threatened again. For me it was the final straw at the time in my catalogue of troubles. My son, a teenager had been feeling ill, saying he had spots before his eyes, and could not see properly, despite all doctor's tests saying they could find nothing wrong. He thought he had a brain tumour. My husband, a solicitor, was winding up his business as a legal aid practitioner, after 12 years of self-employment, and there was considerable worry over a long period of time as to whether bankruptcy was on the cards or not. So, all in all that time of my life was very traumatic for me. About a year after her death, I had my nervous breakdown.

I have always felt sad that my mother missed out on the joys of family life. First she was ill herself as her young children were growing up, but more importantly, she did not see her 3 girls fully grown. Then, she was not around to see our children, her grandchildren. Between us, my two sisters and I have had 6 grandchildren, 2 each, so my mother would have had a ready made family again to surround her with love in her later years. My step-mother had no children of her own, although she had been married once before, so for her, it was lovely to have a ready made family of six grandchildren. Sometimes I look at my children and see my mother in them, particularly my son. And to my daughter I gave the middle name of O'Hara, which was my mother's maiden name. I had hoped in this way that the female line would be represented through the grandchildren. But it has been a source of unhappiness to me that my children did not see their birth grandmother. I have often showed them her photograph, and have talked of her, particularly since the death of their own grandmother. However, I was not aware of this great void in my life until more recent times, I suppose when I had some time to stop and really think about myself and what I had achieved in life.

Chapter 6 - Post-Natal Depression

After the birth of my second child, a delightful little girl, I had nightmares and generally felt totally exhausted. I had had a very quick birth at home, not expected. During the afternoon contractions started about 3.00pm, but I just carried on with my usual tasks. In fact that morning I had been very busy indeed shopping and washing. At quarter to six in the evening I had put my son in the bath, and then the contractions became more severe. Of course I had phoned my husband during the afternoon, and asked him to come home, so he turned up for bath time. We had phoned for an ambulance, at which point I just could not move. When the ambulance turned up, I felt it was too late to go to hospital, so I had my very quick birth at home on the bed. I was on my knees and could not move, so my husband had to cut my underwear off. With a little gas and air for me, my daughter came into the world at 6.10 pm on a Thursday evening. After the birth, a whole medical team turned up from the local hospital, to attend to me, and I was then taken with my baby to the other nearby hospital where my labour had been scheduled. I remember the large ward, a busy place, and how I felt absolutely starving when I arrived and demolished a packet of biscuits and some chocolate. After stitches and five days inside I was allowed to return home. I remember feeling very tired at the time, and this tiredness did not improve. Luckily the grandparents came along to help, and I could take it quite easy for the next two weeks. I found the contrast between my 3 year old big strong son, and my new 6lb baby girl enormous, and genuinely could not cope with the differing demands. It made it more difficult that my daughter was not a good feeder as my son had been, so it was a question of me trying desperately to feed her, to increase her weight and her strength, while she took every opportunity to just nod off asleep. I remember we even set the alarm in the middle of the night, one to wake her up, and the other to breastfeed. That did not work either, so we settled into a routine of feeding on demand for her, rather than routinely feeding every 4 hours as I had done for my son.

The nightmares continued for some two weeks, I think I was worried about the fact that I had given birth so quickly, and it felt a bit like Mary Shelley's Frankenstein, was my baby alright, or had I given birth to a monster. When I was reassured that my daughter was a healthy little girl the nightmares went away, but they were extremely vivid and alarming when I had them. I found a book on post-natal depression which I read as applying to me, even though I was not medically treated for it. Unfortunately my tiredness did not improve for some considerable time, so my husband continued to take my son to the nursery, and collect him after work, until about 6 weeks after the birth, when I felt able to drive the car and cope with my son as well. However, I took on the services of a cleaner, who kept the house nice and tidy for me, and basically I just tried to relax. It did not help that I knew very few mothers at home, because I had returned to work some seven months after my son was born, and was on maternity leave for my daughter's confinement. So, again I was very isolated at home once the grandparents returned home. It is exceedingly difficult to develop a social routine at home, when you have been used to going out to work, especially when you are feeling tired and alone. However, I managed, and I remember enrolling for fitness classes with a crèche when my baby was about 8 weeks old. I went with my sister, who had just given birth to a little girl some six weeks after me.

There was great companionship in that. I returned to work again when my little girl was seven months old, and attending the same nursery as her brother. However, although I enjoyed the work environment again, I found it extremely difficult to manage with my two children and work, so when my daughter was 18 months old I went on a year's child care leave, which in fact turned into my leaving work at that time. My son was four and needed to start at school, so I became a full time mother and was there every day for the two of them. Gradually too, I met friends at the school, one of whom I am still in contact with to this day.

In those days there was very little information around about post-natal depression, so I just managed the best I could. Now there is good widespread knowledge and many ante natal classes deal with the subject. There is also a very good leaflet produced by the Royal College of Psychiatrists, which I would recommend people to read. It is quite clear from the books I have read and the details provided through research that loss of a mother is one of the predisposing factors to post-natal depression, as PND is to development of manic depression. I wish that I had been 'found' by some professional or another in the intervening years, someone who could have helped me cope with my feelings of being a mother without a mother. Unfortunately I did not have any knowledge of the subject myself and also because I was a white, middle-class mother, and presented fairly confidently and did not openly discuss the problems I was experiencing, no one recognised the symptoms for me. Yet, when I took part in a later research project, after my diagnosis of manic depression, one of the questions specifically related to talking about two episodes in my past, when I had felt I needed help. In my case the first one was after the birth of my daughter, during this episode of post natal depression, and the second one was after my miscarriage, some three and a half years later.

Chapter 7 - Miscarriage

My husband set himself up in business when my son was five, and it was a difficult time financially managing on the limited takings he could bring home. I went to help him with the work, and at the same time I became pregnant for the third time, and so left my employment, thinking I would be working with my husband. However, I then had a miscarriage and later decided it would be best if I went out to work again, so I became a locum advice worker, and we took on the services of a young nanny for the children. She was excellent with them, and had lots of energy, but I remember feeling jealous of the time she spent with the children and the attachment they formed for her. My husband had to work long hours for the business and I am afraid I went off the rails a bit for quite a while after my miscarriage. Looking back at the time now, I am sure that my miscarriage and the lack of time and attention paid to the loss, upon the earlier loss of my mother, was the cause of this upset. I became almost manic, and was not thinking straight at all, but I had to keep working, and I stupidly got myself obsessed by someone at work. After this I was quite ill, and I felt very low and depressed, but I had to keep working. We needed the money. Again, only recently have I found the interest and enthusiasm to find out about miscarriage, at the Miscarriage Association, and how it can cause tremendous pain if the loss is not actually acknowledged and dealt with at the time. I did not stop to think for a moment about the loss of my baby, until many years had passed that is. It is now fifteen years since I had my miscarriage and my baby died, but it took me that long to read up about miscarriage. However, within our family, with my husband and our two children, we always talked about the little baby who would have been born, and the age he or she would have been, so that loss became a living part of our immediate family's lives.

Again, after my miscarriage, I decided that it just would not be practical in the circumstances we found ourselves in, to carry on having more children. At the time I accepted this as the most sensible way forward, only later have I had recurring thoughts about it. When we married, my husband and I decided that we would like a family of four children, and things went well until I found life fairly stressful with just two children. I gave up work to concentrate on mothering my children, and found this the most fulfilling part of my existence. However, after my miscarriage, at about nine and a half weeks, for me that was it, my body telling me that it could not cope. Many couples have two children, so it was quite acceptable that I had my two, too. Only my husband and I knew that we really wanted to have a larger family. As my husband was one of eight children, he was used to a number of children together, and he was actually a very natural father, one who loved playing with and instructing his children. As for me, I was the oldest of 3, all girls, and I was not used to being in large groups of children in the same way as my husband. I had to learn about babies when I had my own, whereas my husband David was already an expert nappy changer, and baby bather. Our life just did not work out simply in the sense of being able to concentrate on just parenting at the time, as we had worries with work and the development of business to focus on too. I do not think we were too idealistic in planning ahead for 4 children, but rather, were caught out by the economic circumstances of the time which made child-rearing in the 80's quite a difficult prospect, especially when we did not have local family support.

Chapter 8 - Difficulties of Being a Mother without a Mother

To some extent I now think this is really the crux of my problems, I have found it exceedingly difficult to be a mother without a mother. Recently I have been searching on the internet and found out that there is a wealth of information out there on motherloss, and the pain of losing a mother. In straight logical terms it would seem ridiculous to say that although my mother died some 31 years ago, it is only now that I can logically say I have really missed her being around for the birth of my children and an interest in their and my lives. Yes I have lived my life, but only in the last five or so years have I actually acknowledged to myself the missing mother absent from my life. I took part in a recent survey over the internet which asked me about my feelings bringing up my children without my mother. I read with interest about this work, because it is to be published in book form in 2004 and I think it will make a good read. This research made me realise that my answers were not uncommon; therefore that the interviewer knew the kinds of feelings I had, about how I had been a very overprotective mother, trying to shield my children from the pain which I had gone through. Also it brought home to me the unconscious way I had been living my life as though it might end prematurely, by sort of preparing the children in advance for losing their mother, like I had lost mine. What I mean is, that as I age I have been approaching the age at which my mother died. Every milestone, like the age at which she had her first heart attack, the first child at university, the day my son graduated from university, all of these threw up memories and feelings for me, which I have had to deal with. I must say that my son's graduation was quite traumatic for me, and I felt bound to recount the story to him of the day of my graduation and my mother's subsequent death. Now, as time has passed, the feelings have subsided, and I am preparing for my daughter's graduation next year.

All my married life I have had no living role model to relate to. I substituted my mother-in-law and my step-mother but these were not real flesh and blood mothers. Throughout my children's childhood and youth I have worried about their progress, and been a sort of over-protective carer, yet encouraging them to be independent souls believing they would have to manage on their own as I had had to do. I was anxious about every aspect of my children's care and development, and despite them doing well this did nothing to allay my fears.

My husband has always been close to his mother, particularly I feel since our children were born, and I have felt jealous of this particular bond they shared. I substituted my sister, instead of my mother, but as we were in the same position of bringing up our children together, we could not always help each other satisfactorily, and certainly in the way that a mother would have done. Perhaps because of this close bond my husband has with his mother, I have tried very hard to be close and a loving daughter in law, even at some point telling her that I treated her as my mother. I do not understand all the reasons behind her telling me that she could never be my mother, but her experience as a mature mother of eight children must count for something. And of course, at the time we had that conversation, I was not interested in her reasons for expression of her feelings as much as my own needs. My step-mother had no birth children of her own so she was absolutely delighted to have her step grandchildren, and she, like my mother in law, was an exemplary grandmother. We all loved them too. My two children have been very lucky in respect to their grandparents, as they knew all four grandparents until well on into their mid-teens, which is not a very common experience. But of course my children knew too, especially since the death of their grandmother, that their grandmother was not my own mother. On her death, I had very different feelings and emotions than if it had been my own mother who had died, and I found it particularly hard to relate to my childrens' states of mind. It was not until a friend discussed it with me that I thought it all through and actually sat down and discussed with my children the feelings I had when my mother had died, and how they must be feeling now that their grandmother had died. How complicated family feelings and emotions turn out to be, and yet I thought I could master them! It has been another good five years in passing for me to feel that I am now starting to move out of the mire of feelings that were just pulling me downwards, to trying to acknowledge my feelings and move on.

One of the ways I attempted to deal with these feelings was to seek counselling. It was after I had been diagnosed as manic depressive and the psychiatrist had suggested that I should go on to lithium, I felt I had to seek alternative solutions to my difficulties. I declined the drug offer and continued on Prozac, the anti-depressant I had been on for nearly six years. I sought counselling. I made enquiries at two organisations locally, one offering psycho-analytical approach and the second being Marriage Care where a counsellor would see people either individually or as a couple. At the time a counsellor friend advised me to steer clear of the psychoanalytic approach which could be rather brutal, and so I opted for Marriage Care counselling as a couple. I did not feel that the problem lay just with me; I thought it was best for my husband and I to have counselling together. So we embarked on our ten sessions together – it proved to be a lifesaver. Our counsellor did not take sides, but she helped each of us understand the other better, but particularly to try and work out our own feelings and emotions. For the first time in my life I was able to explore in safety my feelings about my mother's death, and being left alone to cope throughout my adult life except for the support of my husband. It is no wonder that he has felt buffeted by the storms of life when I have been so dependent on him for support and assistance, and neither of us really appreciated the severity of my condition. This counselling gave us a set time each week to just talk about ourselves and our feelings within the security of the confidential room. We were not judged, but each had a time to talk and we listened to each other, sometimes in amazement. I did enjoy the sessions and would have gone on having counselling for a lot longer, but there were time constraints and the counsellor felt we had made sufficient progress for me to cope with life. There was always the proviso that I could return at any time for further counselling sessions alone, should I feel the need, but I have never taken up the option. Our counselling cost £30.00 per hour session which was money well spent, and also made us take responsibility for our treatment.

My psychiatrist does not believe that CBT would help me. CBT is cognitive behavioural therapy, and I have asked on a number of occasions for this treatment. My daughter, who is a psychology student in her third year, believed that this would make a substantial difference to me, and armed with her studied points, both my husband and I asked the psychiatrist on more than one occasion for this for me. The answer was no. I still have the option of seeking private medical treatment through my husband's employee health insurance scheme, but to date I have retained faith with my psychiatrist and his medical opinion. To go forward for private treatment would mean seeking a second opinion, and to me this would undermine the very nature of my treatment which I have been through with the NHS psychiatrist, from my first referral seven years ago to the present day. Besides, at any time I can seek private treatment, providing it is covered through private medical insurance or I can pay privately. At the moment and for the last seven years I have pursued the NHS offering, through my GP.

Again, I took part in another study in 2002, which was being run by the Institute of Psychiatry. I picked up a leaflet in the local library which invited all manic depressives, in beautiful purple and red colours on their leaflet, to take part in research studies to further the understanding of manic depression. So, being completely altruistic and also curious at the same time I made contact with the Institute and offered my experiences as part of their study. I agreed the written terms of reference and made an appointment to go up and see them. Luckily for me the research project had agreed to pay transport costs including necessary taxi fares to their centre, because although I took the tube and arrived at the correct underground station, I then got completely lost and walked in exactly the wrong direction. I think I was quite manic at the time. In desperation, late for my interview, I hailed a taxi and obtained a receipt for the £8.00 costs, knowing that they would be reimbursed; because there is no way that I would have taken a taxi ride without that knowledge. My taxi driver and I had quite a conversation in the ten or so minutes, and I learned that his wife also suffered from manic depression and had done so over 20 years, in so many ways so much more severe than my own condition. He was very interested in the fact that I was taking part in a research project which would eventually lead to better understanding of manic depression and its effect on the family and other carers, which in many cases can be quite devastating. I really enjoyed my interview at the Institute of Psychiatry and the professional nature of the prepared questions, the taped interview and the questionnaires which I was asked to complete. I was pleased to be one of the only people to have pointed out a mistake in one of the questions, so I felt I was not too off the boil! I was asked whether I felt I had been ill in the sense of manic depression prior to the diagnosis being given and of course I had to instance the two times I had felt quite ill, and which I have already written about – one being post-natal depression after the birth of my daughter, and the second being the period of disorientation after my miscarriage. How interesting to be asked for my interpretation of my feelings and my illnesses. Other questions seemed particularly apt to my condition including whether I went on spending sprees, yes I did at the charity shops locally and whether this took me into debt. Luckily, because I have always had to be quite careful about my money, I do not spend huge amounts on credit. But perhaps all those spendaholics are really undiagnosed manic depressives! The interview ended after an hour and three quarters, and a blood test was taken which made it all seem very medical and official. I was also offered the opportunity of follow-up telephone calls if I needed to make any further contact. Because I did think of something on the way home I wrote to the Institute with details of when I had felt nausea when I had had to go to the local hospital for a fibroids scan and at the time I believed they were taking a pregnancy scan. How mixed up can the mind get!! We exchanged a couple of emails and then I felt I had contributed everything I could to their study, and I now await the published results of their research. I feel proud to have been a part of this work and to have made the time and effort to have taken part. Like this written account, you will only learn more if we share it with you.

Again, I have been further contacted by the same Institute to see if I would be willing to take part in another study, about the psychological aspects of manic depression, and I have replied in the affirmative. I do quite enjoy such research anyway, but particularly if I feel it can contribute to a better understanding of a psychiatric condition then it must be worthwhile.

Chapter 9 – My Illness

The amygdala is where fear originates I believe, and of course when I was ill with mania my brain was definitely overloaded with fear and anxiety. I first fell ill 7 years ago when I collapsed in tears and was totally unable to carry on my normal everyday life. I had been exceedingly busy for the previous year, working hard with my husband to sort out his legal aid practice, after he transferred the business from a Kensington office back to our home. I had worked round the clock, only taking time out to do the essentials of washing, shopping, caring for the children, etc. Often we were so tired; the children would make us cups of tea and bring them into the workroom. We had to carry on working, but I also just started to do some physical exercise at the local gym. At first I had got into the exercise, but then I found it more and more difficult, but I persevered. However, after some time I fell ill.

I had not been sleeping well for about 3 nights, and in fact I had been up in the night, sort of raring to go and get on with things which I felt were essential to do. I had bought three little poetry books for my husband and two children, and it was necessary to inscribe them in the middle of the night. For some reason, all sense of time had left me, and maybe I did not even think that I would survive the night. It was imperative that I did what I had to do then and there. This was definitely a bout of mania, now that I can call it by its true name, but at the time, I just thought I had to be up and doing. I remember thinking I might die, but instead of dying like my mother, I thought I should pray, and so I asked my husband to pray with me. Then we managed to get back to sleep.

I remember it was on a Saturday morning, and I felt terrible. The children were not at school, and we were all at home. I remember being quite unable to control my emotions and collapsing in tears. So my sister who lived nearby came round to help. She spent the day with us and that helped. The doctors were alerted by phone, with my sister and my husband, and tranquilisers were prescribed. The emergency prescription was dispensed and I took some pills. It helped to knock me out, which was probably what I needed then and there. My sister moved in to stay the weekend, and she ended up looking after me in the middle of the night when I got up and started wandering around the house, wanting to talk to her about my feelings.

Following a GP appointment there was a referral to the local community psychiatric team, where I was introduced to the psychiatrist and the community psychiatric nurse. As my parents in law had come down to help look after me and the household of my two children, they came along to the appointment with us, and were able to input their thoughts on a written sheet of paper too. My husband and I were both interviewed separately and together. I remember vividly thinking it was not me who was ill but my husband and that surely everyone could see that. We had all been under a lot of strain with working from home for the last year or so, and I had had to deal with the builders working on a loft extension who ran off in the middle of the job. Family matters had been quite demanding too, so it was not surprising that we ended up at the psychiatrist. However, it all seemed rather unreal to me, and I sat there in the psychiatrist's waiting room smiling away, thinking all would be revealed.

This however was just the start of the process and these long years later I am only now starting to feel that I am on top of my illness and not that it is ruling me. For nearly 7 years I have been up and down, sometimes feeling well, other times feeling so depressed I did not want to get out of bed, and sometimes thought there was no point in me living. I have suffered extreme agitation and various side-effects from the prescribed drugs, but did not know whether they were symptoms of the illness of problems associated with drug-taking. I tried to understand what was happening to me, but it is a difficult thing to take charge of your mind when you are experiencing mental health difficulties. My mind tended to drift, in and out of a consciously and unconsciously controlled state, and really I had no idea how I would be feeling the next day, often the next hour, or even the next few minutes. My agitation was great, and I felt very anxious about everything. I regularly thought that my close family members would come to grief and have an accident, and I would be constantly checking up on where everyone was, and how they were. I could not settle or relax until they returned home, only to go through the same round of worries the next day when they set off again.

I had to teach myself that no news is good news, and try to stop these thoughts going round my head. But of course I also worried about myself and particularly car journeys, thinking there would be an accident. I did not worry about train, boat or plane journeys, because there the control was taken away from me. But with driving our car, I was constantly worried about the thought of an accident, and it spoilt my enjoyment on any trip or outing. May I add that I have always had this worry about car journeys, since I started driving myself, and it is much worse for me if I go in the car driven by someone else. Of course the other side of worry is that you get to the point where you decide the best thing to do is not to show you are worried, because of the reaction you get from others. Consequently I have found myself becoming rather aloof to my family and I think I have lost that spontaneous nature of talking, or phoning and speaking to them that I used to have. Now it all seems so much more calculated, and I need to prepare myself before speaking, or picking up the phone, so that I come over as OK.

There have been different regimes of medications throughout the years, and also the twice when I tried to wean myself off the anti-depressants before I realised that I couldn't cope. Sometimes I have felt really drugged up and thought the power of the medication was too strong for me to be able to do anything. At other times, of course prior to my diagnosis of manic depression when I was on anti-depressants alone – some five years - my mind would be wandering off and my concentration appalling. So what with anxiety, mania and depression I have experienced a right mixed bag of emotions and feelings. It must have been really difficult for my family and friends to know how to cope with me, and in the end it is particularly my immediate family of my husband and two children who have really suffered. Their story is next. As regards my friends, I am afraid that many of the relationships have really deteriorated and it is only the ones who persistently made an effort to keep in contact with me who have survived, either because they understood something about mental health problems or they themselves wanted to keep up the contact. In addition I have made more contacts with other people who have shared my experience of mental health problems and illness, so I have broadened my circuit of friendship types.

Chapter 10 - My Husband In His Own Words And How The Family Has Coped With My Illness

I asked my husband if he would write a chapter for me on how he has managed to cope with me and my illness and what sort of an effect it has all had on the family. He readily agreed. Here you are – these are his words.

"Well, it's so difficult for me to say. I always thought that you had suffered from post-natal depression which never stopped, but merged into all of the ordinary difficulties of a young family. But one day, years later, without warning, a terrible thing happened. Within a few days you lost your wits. At first I thought it would go away like a bad mood, but in the end there was a complete breakdown. All the doctors could do, or would do, was to prescribe pills which laid you out flat. After three months of anxiety, and friends and relatives simply watching over you, the doctor said it was quite simple, it was depressive illness, and six months of Prozac would cure it. This was rather startling because it seemed the opposite of reality. After fifteen years of depression you were anything but depressed. Crazy maybe, but not depressed. It worked. The fears and strange ideas were gone. But in their place the happy pill did not bring back the old you. After six months, the Prozac stopped and the tears started with swarms of anxieties. Then back to Prozac, this time for ever. This did not work either. Eventually, despite Prozac, there was another breakdown, with wild fancies and irrational behaviour. So this time it was anti-psychotic drugs, giving an unnatural calm. Nothing seemed to bring back your former self. This time the description was manic depression and a prospect of seeking out the right cocktail of chemicals to restore some elusive brain chemical balance. Two further episodes lead to further refinements. Talking cures and cognitive therapy and anything other than drugs was dismissed as ineffective.

All this time we carried on as best as we could, hoping that living a normal and healthy life would somehow lead to a normal and healthy mind. We did yoga and exercise, went swimming and did country walks. We went on adventurous holidays and enjoyed more time together as the children went off to university. The worst fears of institutionalisation were never realised, but getting back to normality was always elusive. You escaped from one set of fears only to acquire another. You recovered one facility only to lose another. It was like trying to catch bubbles; it was easy to question what normality is in the first place. It led to dependence and a loss of independence, which was both flattering and daunting to me.

It seems strange that the breakdown resulted in a fundamental change in the dynamics of the family, just at the point that they would have changed anyway. As the children approached independence, your role as the centre of the family was coming to an end, and my role as the head of a family business with long, laborious hours away from the family, was also coming to an end. The point where the doctor was called for was when you started shouting in the middle of the night, demanding that a priest be called. This woke the children. You told them that their father had gone mad and I told them that you had suffered a breakdown.

They looked from one to the other and back again, bewildered. After that, it was a house of sickness, with the breakdown treated as an illness. This was true in as much as you had lost a faculty, like walking or talking. But there was no diagnosis, no cure, no accident, no injury, no germ or virus, only palliatives, which made you feel bad, but made you calm.

I had no idea where it would lead. I went to the doctor to make an appointment for you and then persuaded you to go. You did not accept you were ill, but more or less acquiesced in your treatment. I was horrified by the state you had been reduced to and moved by compassion for your plight, which you found very frightening. Our daughter asked her school chums to see if any of them had any similar experience which could give her a guide to her own fate. She found such a thing was not at all rare and other friends had been through much the same themselves. She concluded you would get better, but not completely better. Our son, who had his own difficulties in coping with the sixth form, where he was floundering, tried to ignore it all, but he was obviously deeply moved.

In a curious way our daughter's observations proved correct. You saw the psychiatrist after 3 months. He was always rather taciturn and did not speculate about the future, but believed the condition would be controlled, whatever that might be. The months turned into years and the illness has not gone away, but complete breakdown has become only a threatening presence in the background, which has come back only occasionally to be been beaten off by prescriptions of pills. Although you are often pessimistic of your progress and of your ability to recover, I do feel that you are advancing. I miss your drive and energy, but I am glad that the anger which seemed to have come with the post-natal depression has long gone. It seems that you could have the best of both worlds, the energy without the anger. Surely they are not inseparable twins.

In any case there is real pleasure in caring for somebody who needs it. Perhaps this is how you felt towards your children when they were helpless babies. Certainly I never expected this turn of events, which came as a complete surprise to me. So, no doubt the future will also be a complete surprise. There has been so much that is positive in this experience. I am impatient for the day when you overcome this illness, but if it ever does pass, I will remember the good side of this frightening experience."

Chapter 11 – Marriage and Bringing Up My Two Children

Let me put the context of my marriage and children into the perspective of my illness. After I finished at university in Edinburgh, I moved south to start work. I had quite a good time really making new contacts and friends in a new area, and soon met up with my husband to be, David Brocklesby. We went out together, and ended up after about six months spending our spare time together. When I undertook my post-graduate course and had a placement in London, David would sometimes come up at weekends, and we spent a lot of time writing and speaking on the phone. So, after some two further years in Guildford, Surrey, we moved to London together and set up in a flat in St. John's Wood. We managed later to get an unfurnished flat over in Hammersmith, West London, from which we got married in 1978.

Our wedding on Saturday 17th June took place at Holy Trinity Church in Olympia, and we held our reception by the River Thames near the Hammersmith Bridge, in a pub overlooking the water. It was a lovely day, and one which we had arranged virtually all on our own. David and I had set the day, we booked the church and the reception and David designed the wedding invitation card, in a lovely sepia. It showed the picture of two people embracing and comforting each other. David had a stag night and I spent the evening quietly at my sister's house in Fulham. Relatives came from Scotland and Banbury, and friends from London and further a field. My sister came with me to buy my lovely Edwardian lace wedding dress from the Kings Road, just as I had spent the day shopping with her to find her outfit. I had something old, something new, something borrowed and something blue, either from my sister or which I bought myself. David and I arranged the gold rings together, and we ordered the wedding cake from our local bakery, with an additional tier for the occasion of baptism of our first child. We were thoroughly involved in all aspects of our wedding and the ceremony, and so felt in control of the situation. Our families came to enjoy the day and my father, as is traditional paid for the reception. After the success of the occasion we left by Rolls Royce for the airport, for our honeymoon in Corfu, Greece.

Christopher, our son was born in February 1980, 20 months after our wedding, following a spell of some weeks in hospital for me on bed rest. He was well and truly wanted and we adored him. Life seemed perfect with our golden haired baby boy. I enjoyed looking after him, breastfeeding every 4 hours, and he grew and grew. We stayed initially with my sister in Fulham, as we had been homeless really at the time of his birth, attempting to move from our unfurnished flat to a little one bedroom flat we just managed to buy in Hammersmith. I regularly had to go and do painting duties in the flat prior to our moving in. So, although we were keen to get the place of our own, it was quite hard work doing the renovation required, at the same time as looking after my son. But somehow we managed, and then moved in when Christopher was some 4 months old. When he was 7 months old I found a child minder and I had to return to work to help pay for our living expenses. I found it really hard having to leave my baby every morning at the child minder, but he was well looked after. At 18 months he transferred to a lovely little private nursery and I continued working feeling happier that he was now in regular contact with lots of other little people. This life continued for quite some time, we moved to a three bed roomed house in Wandsworth, and then I went on maternity leave and had my daughter Elizabeth in December 1982. Life became more complicated with two children to look after and I found it very difficult trying to balance the needs of the family and cope with being a mother and a wife. I initially suffered from post-natal depression and terrible nightmares after the birth of my daughter, and the tiredness and the worry continued for months afterwards. I think it was really me feeling that I could not manage so simply any more. One child fitted in to the schedule and the way of life quite easily without that much disruption, whereas two children required complete adaptation to a family life. Although my father and step-mother came down to help me initially for the first two weeks, which was a great help, after their departure, I was left to my own devices, and found the challenge rather too much for me. There was no one else to help, so during the day, David took our son Christopher to nursery and I spent the day looking after my daughter. I needed to recover, so I spent a lot of time resting with her. Only after about 6 weeks was I able to use the car and take my son myself to nursery and continue to look after Lizzie during the day. The days seemed so busy, and I felt permanently exhausted. However, after about 4-5 months I did recover somewhat. We had a very restful holiday in

France where we enjoyed the peaceful surroundings of a seaside holiday home, and then I returned to go back to work, with both my children at the nursery.

I never really managed to settle into this pattern of work again. It was really too much for me. So, after about 8-9 months I went on a year's child care leave. I don't know how I lasted so long, because I was constantly rushing, I started to feel stressed, and I was always worried about my work and suffered palpitations and chest pains. So, I was glad to stop work, even though the money had been extremely important in setting up home in our new 3 bed roomed house in Wandsworth. My son at this time was ready to start school and my daughter and I would find activities to do together, including things like mother and baby swimming lessons, and the local playgroups. However, Elizabeth had problems with eczema, and so we had a number of hospital appointments to deal with, including special elimination diets, all in an effort to try and cut out the causes of her eczema. This helped a little, but we embarked on learning how to cook healthy wholesome meals, which continued throughout her childhood.

I became a full-time mother until it was necessary for me to return to work again, after I had my miscarriage, and my husband was setting up his new legal aid practice in Kensington. I employed a full-time nanny and I did more advice work in London bureaux. I think however, that my emotions were really mixed up with my miscarriage and my immediate feelings that there would be no more children. My husband and I found it a great strain, and to some extent we lost our way. I went off the rails, and looking back now, I see this time as a warning for my later breakdown. However, I did not go to the doctor, there was no offer of counselling after a miscarriage, no one talked to me about it at all. I was just left to get on with life, being a mother and looking after my two children. The miscarriage itself involved an overnight stay in hospital and a D & E operation, and then all was back to normal. Nowadays I believe that in miscarriage mothers are left to miscarry naturally, which seems a more healthy process. There is no hospital and surgical intervention – therefore you probably would not think of it as so much of a final solution. With things happening naturally in their own good time, you would have time to adjust. There would be no drugs with the anaesthetic and no removal to hospital. In my case there was no advantage in being removed to hospital, because I did not receive any care for my miscarriage at all. In fact it was all treated in a completely matter of fact way, and there was no reference at all to my baby, and the loss of my baby. To me I think this was just another example of the alienation of motherhood in the hospital system. At the time I just accepted it, because I knew no different. Now, I realise how much more sensitively I could have been helped. We live and learn.

Then life continued with our two children and we felt we were complete as a family of four. We worked hard, looked after the children as our priority and took them on exciting holidays. By this time I had given up outside work for good, and took in secretarial work. We managed to move to a larger house in Wandsworth, and I set up my own business working from home, so that I could be around at all times for my two children, now aged 4 and 7. On the whole this was quite a good time for us, the only problem being that my husband had to work such long hours to make his business pay. I managed at home well with the children, and the three of us used to do a lot together during the week. After school we would go to the various activities around for children, like the family gym, like the family computer class, like the after school swimming, and then there was the arts and drama, including ballet and acting classes, not to mention the various guitar, or violin lessons. I became an active chauffeur after school, and was fully involved in all my children's activities. For my day job I ran my secretarial business, doing computer and word processing work for the various clients I attracted through local advertising. The business proved fairly profitable as well, which was just as well because the late 80's was a period of high interest rates, and our mortgage became absolutely extortionate. But we just managed. My husband was building up his legal practice, with the help of his sister, and I was based at home, looking after the children and running my own firm, with which I was fairly adaptable. Like in the holidays, I did not take on any work at all, and was around for the children, and together we enjoyed doing family activities, and visiting grandparents. We always made time for our family holidays, and they were always exciting for our children.

Then, when the children were both teenagers, we decided we had to move to a cheaper house because my husband's business was going through a very difficult time. We moved, and settled the children in. Then my son was having difficulty with his school work and kept telling us his eyesight was deteriorating, and despite medical tests we could find nothing wrong. My step-mother died after a stroke and about 12 weeks illness. We attempted to go on holiday before this, but it was very much coloured by the worry over my son, and my step-mother. At this time my husband had closed his London offices and had moved his work back to the house, and we were very busy trying to cope with the demands upon us. Then, I'm afraid I had my nervous breakdown, and I became subject to medical attention and was under the care of a psychiatrist.

Chapter 12 - The Role of My Psychiatrist

I have many letters from the psychiatrist to myself, as copies of the letters he has written to my GP to keep her in touch with my condition. I think this is a particularly useful way of reflecting back on the actual appointment with the psychiatrist, because it is all a process of care. The psychiatrist is the key worker here in partnership with the patient. It is essential that the patient receives copies of psychiatrist's letters, to be fully informed. However, at times when I have been really ill, it has been important for my husband to read these letters, and he would accompany me on the appointments to see the psychiatrist. At first, I had a care plan, and would regularly see the community psychiatric nurse, either at the hospital, or in my own home.
A couple of times I had corresponded with my psychiatrist by email when I had wanted to check up on a point in one of the letters, or to ask him a further question. My psychiatrist said that I was one of only two patients who had ever used the email facility to correspond with him, and that he found it quite helpful, just like I did, to clear up any questions. I have been discharged from care in the past, only to be re-referred by my GP when I had another episode. Late in 2003, the psychiatrist hoped to discharge me from his care at the next routine appointment, and he did discuss this with me at the previous session. I see no reason why I need to continually see the psychiatrist now that my medication has stabilised, and I can get my prescriptions from my GP. However, re-referral is always a possibility should my condition change or should I have another bad attack. But I am confident

now that I have some insight into my condition, that I will be able to self-manage it now myself, with the help of the prescribed medication. I wrote a poem about this called 'Doctor and Patient' and you will be able to read it in the section on Poems for Mental Health. I gave my psychiatrist a copy of the first version of my book, actually via another psychiatrist who reviewed me on the last appointment.

Chapter 13 - Medication and Self Help

Throughout the years, I have remained on prescribed medication, except for one or two spells where I tried to wean myself off. It just did not work. I could not manage without medication. When I was first ill a tranquiliser was prescribed, and then that was replaced by an anti-psychotic drug and an anti-depressant. So although the anti-psychotic was then deemed unnecessary, until I had a relapse, it is now felt that I need to be on both an anti-depressant and an anti-psychotic, although the latter is a low dose.

It does not seem to me that we can just say that we do not want medication, because when we have the correct drug and prescription, it does seem to make me feel better. So we need to build on to the medication and try various self-help remedies too to improve our condition. Exercise, diet, lifestyle all play their part, along with the attempt to live as normal a life as possible with friendships, work/life balance, and development. Prior to my illness I was always able to work, but since then I have had difficulty with coping with work, so at the moment I am attempting to deal with this. My psychiatrist thinks I am capable of work, and in fact encourages me to work. In fact it is my low self-esteem and worry about being able to do the work that causes me the problem. I find myself making excuses to myself. Even so it is a very real problem as to whether or not we can find work which suits us after a mental illness. To work on this problem of lack of self confidence I enrolled in an adult education class which helped us over a ten week period to look at all aspects of our behaviour in dealing with situations in an assertive way. I found it particularly helpful to work within a small group of like-minded individuals who all had taken the course to work on this aspect of their self, and through our exercise programme I learned to grow in confidence. I also bought a couple of books on confidence building which served to reinforce what I had learned at class. To a large extent I think confidence depends on whether we have a network of supportive friends around us, as in my experience, my illness led to social withdrawal, loss of outside work and gradually less self-confidence. It is thus important to deal with this aspect of self-help, and to work again towards social integration and increasing social contact in the job market.

After a particularly distressing relapse where I had become quite ill with psychosis, my social contacts and confidence plummeted to zero. I was in tears the whole time, and I just felt that I was no use to anyone at all. After stabilising my medication I was introduced to the Occupational Therapist of the team whose job was to help with social integration through work or work experience. I was desperate to try for paid work, but actually it was totally unrealistic. So the OT suggested that I try some voluntary work. This was a brilliant suggestion. I had often in the past worked with volunteers, and in fact had offered my time and services occasionally to a voluntary group, so I knew the sector. I was introduced to a specialist service operating in our area, and the co-ordinator worked specifically with people with mental health difficulties who wished to do voluntary work. She had built up a small network of organisations in the area which would offer placements to people like myself. So after an exploratory meeting where I was made to feel very welcome at this placement service, and gently introduced to the services offered, through a welcome cup of coffee, I had an interview with my local charity, Crimestoppers. I had to provide my CV, and then received an offer of voluntary work two days a week. It was all placed on an organised official level with a letter offering work and a confidentiality statement to sign, so I felt it was an achievement to have arrived at this point. This gave me confidence too. So I have now been working in a voluntary capacity two days a week at my local charity office over the last year. I have been doing a variety of tasks and have been instructed on the use of computer programmes, so I feel I have learned a lot of useful things, as well as had the benefit of working in the social context of an office setting. Even though it was a great effort initially for me to get in to work, I have managed it apart from a five week spell where I was unwell, and now it has become routine for me to go to work two days a week, so I have made definite progress and recovered some of my confidence in practice. I have now also signed on with a local secretarial and employment agency to do paid work and I have completed two very part-time, short term appointments. Initially I will work part-time, on occasion, unless something suitable comes up, and then hopefully increase again to longer hours when I feel able to do so. I have done this kind of work as a secretary before, so it will not be anything too difficult for me to deal with. For those who need retraining there are often courses laid on and it is worth finding out what is available in your area.

One of the main difficulties I have had over the years since my illness first occurred is maintaining friendships, so that my social contacts have become more restricted, and I have become increasingly dependent at times on my husband. He has coped amazingly with it, as you will have read in his account of how the family has coped, but no one person can be the only supportive figure in someone's life. We all need others in our life. Now when I was very ill, it was too much of an effort even to go out at all except just to the local shops for the food for the evening meal, and sometimes even that was too much for me. It is at times like this that we need support services in the local community. I did contact the local group who offered voluntary visiting for people with mental health problems, but I found that I was ineligible because I did not live alone. I remember feeling very disappointed at the time, and really quite isolated, but I did not know where else to turn. Friends and contacts do not want to hear about your mental health difficulties, even though you may want to talk about them. It is a vicious circle, even though you are ill you may look well like I did, and no one knows the trauma that is going on in your mind, or the constant thoughts that may be racing through your head. The local community looks such a busy place and everybody is going about their daily business, but because you are inward looking you have no one to talk to. I even wrote a poem about this because it struck me so intensely, and you will find this also in my Poems For Mental Health. I was not referred to any of the local services for people with mental health problems probably because I was not one of the priority needs as I did not live alone, but I knew of the various centres which were open, like day centres and drop-in centres. They were not what I wanted to visit. I just wanted someone to come into my home to talk to me and make me feel that someone out there actually cared about me and wanted to know how I was managing. Appointments at the local hospital for out-patient appointments do not serve that purpose. Perhaps what I am talking about is a local buddy scheme for people with mental health difficulties, for those who are isolated at home. It is most likely a temporary need, and once we are over the worst may no longer be necessary, but it could speed up the rehabilitation process and help us not to feel so alone.

One of the other factors that are worth raising though is the side effects of prescribed medication. I have been reading a book, 'Psychiatry, The Ultimate Betrayal' by Bruce Wiseman, and I found listed the various side effects of the commonly used drug Prozac. I don't think in all the 6-7 years I was on Prozac anyone actually told me about the side effects, although I always read the instruction leaflet that came from the manufacturers of the drug. Here is the long list of side effects, many of which I recognise. I can honestly say that I am pleased to no longer be on this prescribed drug. 'According to psychiatrist David L Richman, one study of this drug reported mild and short-lasting effects in these percentages: nausea (25%), nervousness

(21%), insomnia (19%), headache (17%), tremors (16%), anxiety (15%), drowsiness (14%), dry mouth (14%), excessive sweating (12%), and diarrhoea (10%). The full list of side effects, as listed in the PDR (Physician's Desk Reference), Family Guide to Prescription Drugs, are as follows:-

More common side effects may include: Abnormal dreams, agitation, anxiety, bronchitis, chills, diarrhoea, dizziness, drowsiness and fatigue, hay fever, inability to fall or stay asleep, increased appetite, lack or loss of appetite, light-headedness, nausea, nervousness, sweating, tremors, weakness, weight loss, yawning.

Less common side effects may include: Abnormal ejaculation, abnormal gait, abnormal stoppage of menstrual flow, acne, amnesia, apathy, arthritis, asthma, belching, bone pain, breast cysts, breast pain, brief loss of consciousness, bursitis, chills and fever, conjunctivitis, convulsions, dark, tarry stool, difficulty in swallowing, dilation of pupils, dimness of vision, dry skin, ear pain, eye pain, exaggerated feeling of well-being, excessive bleeding, facial swelling due to fluid retention, fluid retention, hair loss, hallucinations, hangover effect, hiccups, high or low blood pressure, hives, hostility, impotence, increased sex drive, inflammation of the oesophagus, inflammation of the gums, inflammation of the stomach lining, inflammation of the tongue, inflammation of the vagina, intolerance of light, involuntary movement, irrational ideas, irregular heartbeat, jaw or neck pain, lack of muscle coordination, low blood pressure upon standing, low blood sugar, migraine headache, mouth inflammation, neck pain and rigidity, nosebleed, ovarian disorders, paranoid reaction, pelvic pain, pneumonia, rapid breathing, rapid heartbeat, ringing in the ears, severe chest pain, skin inflammation, skin rash, thirst, twitching, uncoordinated movements, urinary disorders, vague feeling of bodily discomfort, vertigo, weight gain.

Rare side effects may include: Abortion, antisocial behaviour, blood in urine, bloody diarrhoea, bone disease, breast enlargement, cataracts, colitis, coma, deafness, decreased reflexes, dehydration, double vision, drooping of eyelids, duodenal ulcer, enlarged abdomen, enlargement of liver, enlargement or increased activity of thyroid gland, excess growth of course hair on face, chest, etc., excess uterine or vaginal haemorrhage, extreme muscle tension, eye bleeding, female milk production, fluid accumulation and swelling in the head, fluid build up in larynx and lungs, gallstones, glaucoma, gout, heart attack, hepatitis, high blood sugar, hysteria, inability to control bowel movements, increased salivation, inflammation of eyes and eyelids, inflammation of fallopian tubes, inflammation of testes, inflammation of the gallbladder, inflammation of the small intestine, inflammation of tissue below skin, kidney disorders, lung inflammation, menstrual disorders, mouth sores, muscle inflammation or bleeding, muscle spasms, painful sexual intercourse for women, psoriasis, rashes, reddish or purplish spots on the skin, reduction of body temperature, rheumatoid arthritis, seborrhoea, shingles, skin discoloration, skin inflammation and disorders, slowing of heart rate, slurred speech, spitting blood, stomach ulcer, stupor, suicidal thoughts, taste loss, temporary cessation of breathing, tingling sensation around the mouth, tongue discoloration and swelling, urinary tract disorders, vomiting blood, yellow eyes and skin.'

Help! And I existed for so many years on this drug without being aware that some of the problems I was experiencing could have been due to the drug I was taking. Yet how come some people think we should become a Prozac nation?

Chapter 14 - Exercise Diet and Lifestyle

My psychiatrist suggested that I might benefit from going to the Diet and Lifestyle group which operated on a Monday in the local outpatient clinic of the psychiatric hospital. I agreed to go along and attended regularly although there were only two other participants on my course. I did not have a key worker which made me stand out from the start; however, I stuck with it, and learned a certain amount from mere participation in the group learning. Here is a copy of the report which was issued to us, at the wind up of the course, at the same time as we gave our evaluation of what we had learned. I learned a bit more again by re-reading the information before retyping the report for this book.

'The Healthy Lifestyle Group is a forum for group discussion about food and exercise to motivate for changing your lifestyle to a more healthy way of living. The duration was made up of eight sessions, and provided an insight into
- Nutrition by Nikki (OT student)
- Self-esteem and motivation by Anita (social worker)
- Physical health by Simon (CPN)
- Diet by Theresa (Dietician)
- Physical activity by Alison (Health and Fitness Advisor)
- Medication by Sanjaya (CPN)

This handout is to remind you about some of the issues covered in these sessions in hope that you will continue to use this knowledge to make subtle changes. Caution must be taken not to make big sudden changes to diet or exercise, but start gradually.

THANK YOU for participating and showing commitment to the group, that alone is evidence that you wish to live a healthier lifestyle.

We wish you good luck in enjoying good health

Coordinators: Sanjaya Warnatilake CPN
               Anita Michelsen SW

Nutrition:

Carbohydrates supply the body with most of its energy. They should be in the form of complex carbohydrates, such as brown rice, wholemeal bread, wholemeal pasta, wholegrain cereals, seeds, nuts, beans and lentils.

The majority of nutrition has been removed in refined food, such as white bread, jam, cakes and sweets.

The body needs some fats/oils. The more healthy kind of fat is mono-saturated vegetable oil, such as olive oil, nuts and Omega 3 Oils as in some seafood.

Fibre can be found in bran cereals, as well as in fruits and vegetables.

Diet:

A balanced diet should ensure sufficient vitamins and minerals, hence, no need for supplements.

Fruits and vegetables are good sources of carbohydrates and are low in fat. Daily recommendation is five portions of fruit for men and four portions of fruit for women.

Grill, bake, or stir-fry instead of pan-frying. If frying, add no more than a teaspoon of oil.

Drink up to two litres of water a day. Teas and coffees contain caffeine, which is a stimulant drug, and it is debatable as to whether this should be counted as part of the daily liquid intake.

Avoid fizzy drinks, and remember that a litre of fruit juice may contain sugar levels equal to three and a half Mars bars. Instead, replace with sugar-free drinks.

Alcohol is fattening, but it has been argued that one glass a day in moderation is healthy.

Dairy products, such as low-fat yoghurts, are ideal for dressings and sauces, and can replace cream. Also, cottage cheese is very healthy and can be used in salads instead of dressings. Drink semi-skimmed or skimmed milk instead of full-fat. Alternatively, drink goats or Soya milk. Drink or eat one to two dairy products a day.

<u>Physical health:</u>

Protein helps growth and build muscles, repairs the body and fights infection. Good sources are fish (Omega 3 oils for example as in kippers), poultry, eggs, and lean meat (fat removed) and beans.

The type of fat consumed has consequences on the overall health. There are some good fats, but saturated oils are unhealthy. Fat gives energy and contains certain vitamins, but if consumed more than needed the fat will be deposited in our body; and as a result may lead to weight gain. Weight gain may have adverse effects on the overall well-being, i.e. Psychological and physical health.

Sources of calcium help nails, hair and bones, and can be found in water and dairy produce.

Our bodies are made of over 60% of water, and dehydration is often caused through sweating, breathing and elimination of waste. It is therefore important to drink a lot; recommended up to 2 litres of water a day.

Fibre may help prevent development of diabetes, gallstones, constipation and other gut disorders, including peptic ulcers, as well as lower cholesterol, dissolve unwanted clots in blood, and eliminate waste.

Alcohol is fattening, and other side-effects include damages to heart and liver, as well as destroying brain cells.

Exercise reduces the risk of heart disease, boosts the immune system, and improves sleep patterns; as well it may help prevent osteoporosis, which is common in menopausal women.

Exercise

The natural man ate when there was food, and starved until next meal. Also, throughout history the human being has worked physically hard. Today, the modern man tends to drive rather than walk, and utilise modern accessories to carry out tasks. Accordingly, there is a need for making an effort to carry out regular exercise.

The recommendation is 30 minutes five times a week. To process more oxygen more efficiently throughout the body a brisk-walking one bus stop further or cycling is advised.

Fresh air and sunshine helps on mood, and a brisk walk in the park is a good form for recharging energy. Also, recreation and rest, in particular regular sleep patterns, may prevent illness and stress.

Laughter is a wonderful way to combine facial exercise with relaxation, and it is healthy for heart and mind.

Strength type of activities include carrying shopping, climbing stairs, gardening and housework. Flexibility type of activities include dancing, swimming and yoga.

Medication

Medication may increase appetite and thirst, therefore it is important to be aware of what you eat and drink.

Medication affects the metabolism, which is the way you may digest the food and drinks you consume, and thus, how much of it the body absorbs.

Newer anti-psychotic medication has less traditional side-effects (for example, stiffness of limbs), but increases the risk of weight gain, whereas newer anti-depressants has less risk of weight gain.

The type and dose of medication may have an impact on weight gain, as well as, the time of day it is taken. However NEVER change the dose, type or routine without consulting your Care Coordinator, as this may be detrimental to your physical and mental health.

Remember that each individual may experience different side-effects, and that not all people put on weight just because there is an added risk in regards to particular medication. It can be caused by too poor a diet, and too little exercise.

The golden rule is to balance regular exercise with good diet, and remember that medication is prescribed to make you better.

Self-Esteem

People with low self-esteem may feel less motivated,
and therefore, do not take proper care of themselves,
i.e. eat too much, or not take care of personal hygiene.
Sometimes, people may eat and drink for comfort.

Loss of self-esteem is sometimes a consequence of
some other problem, which causes distress and
disruption in the person's life.

Combating self-critical thoughts by raising awareness,
and viewing yourself more positively.

One good exercise is to stand in front of the mirror each
morning, and say out loud one good thing about
yourself before starting the day with a healthy
breakfast.

What matters most is how you see yourself – remember
that picture of a little cat looking in a mirror and seeing
the reflection of a lion!" This all ties in with the self-
confidence and increasing self-esteem classes which I
had already attended by this time in the course.

One of the very useful individual sessions was that of
the effects of medication on weight gain. It transpires
that anti-depressants have a low effect on weight gain,
but that some of the anti-psychotics do have an effect.
Here is some of the information, because it is worth
knowing about. Printed from the Psychopharmacology
of antipsychotic, no change or weight loss from
Loxapine and Molindone; increasing likelihood of

weight gain are: Ziprasidone (the least weight gain), Thiothixene, Fluphenazine, Haloperidol, Risperidone, Chlorpromazine, Sertindole, Quetiapine, Thioridazine, Olanzapine, Zotepine, Clozapine (the greatest weight gain). What affects a patient's weight? Medication may affect weight, because of increased hunger, increased thirst, metabolic changes, reduced activity and feeling well. But we were also taught that everyone can manage their weight! So Risperidone comes nearer the least weight gain side, which is good news for me. Also I was pleased to see that both Prozac and Efexor were low sedation and no weight gain reported.

Chapter 15 - Anxiety

Now that I am on an anxiety reducing anti-depressant, Efexor XL, I feel less anxiety. But for most of my life I have been a fairly anxious person, even though I thought I was calm and presented a calm front to the world. I think that sometimes I am calm but I could become agitated and anxious. When I first became ill with depression 7 years ago, I was put on to Prozac, an anti-depressant, and had a little Risperdal, an anti-psychotic, for a few weeks, but I did not realise at the time that I was anxious. It is only as the years have gone by that I have read a little about anxiety and now believe that is what I suffer from. I remember a huge panic attack one day when my husband was going to take me swimming. We had gone to the pool and bought our tickets, when suddenly I felt that I could not go in the water. I remembered reading an article in the previous week in the local paper about an elderly man who had had a heart attack in the water there, and subsequently died. My feeling was that it would be me next if I went in to swim. So, we did not go swimming, but instead went for a little walk outside on the grassy area near the building. My heart started to pound, and I was exceedingly worried. I had never had this feeling before. I thought it must be my nerves and worry, but also at the same time I wondered if I might be having a heart attack, as my mother had done all those years before. After all I was nearly 50 and she had her first attack when she was that age. So, we kept walking, but slowly and I described my feelings to my husband, of how my chest was throbbing, and I felt weak. Then my legs started to go wobbly too, and so we took to the car to go home. By the time we got home the condition had improved a bit, but I went for a rest until I had recovered. I don't know what had brought it on, except that this was just before I became seriously ill, and I think it was just a reflection of how my body and mind were feeling – totally exhausted. It was a really scary feeling having a panic attack because you feel the physical symptoms are so real, and naturally tend to think in terms of a physical condition as a cause. Of course, as I managed to carry on walking without collapsing in a heap, or feeling intense pain in my chest or upper arms, I believed that it must be alright, in the sense that I could not be having a heart attack, which for me would have been the worst scenario. But I had explained my feelings to my husband, so that if I did collapse he would know to take me to hospital where they could investigate heart trouble.

Since then I have experienced many symptoms of anxiety, but it is not until I found a booklet produced by MIND called 'Understanding Anxiety' that I realised that was what I was suffering from. I mean that I had suffered jelly legs, I had felt nauseous, and light-headed, and I had felt really agitated, and not been able to settle to anything, because of a jittery feeling and breathing difficulties. For a long time, when I went out on a walk I had the feeling that I would perhaps collapse, with my legs giving way underneath me, and all the time I was walking my legs would be shaky and cause me to feel very tired. My whole body would be tense and I would be preoccupied in my mind that perhaps my body would not make it, so that although I wanted to go on a walk to improve my fitness level, it was as though my body was fighting against that. For me exercise has never been easy, so it has been a constant battle to try and summon up the enthusiasm to want to go out walking to improve my fitness level anyway. At other times, again my body has really fought against wanting to do exercise; when e.g. just before an exercise class I would feel panicky as to whether I could actually do the exercise in the class. I would get shaky and light headed. Other symptoms of anxiety for me have been teeth and jaw grinding, and my head spinning with thoughts. However, in reading this booklet it has helped me understand my anxiety and how it manifests itself in physical symptoms, which other people have experienced as well, so this has been quite reassuring for me. I realise that I am not alone, and that others have felt the same nausea, and jelly legs as I have experienced. What are the effects of anxiety? 'Anxiety affects body and mind. Increased muscular tension can cause discomfort and headaches. Breathing rapidly may make you feel light-headed and shaky, and give you pins and needles. Rising blood pressure can make you more aware of a pounding heart. Changes to the blood supply affecting the digestive system may also cause nausea and sickness.' I do recommend this useful little booklet to anyone who thinks they may be suffering from anxiety.

There is great similarity between physical and psychological pain. For someone who has a back ache they may take to their beds thinking that bed rest is the best thing, whereas in fact I understand the best thing is mobility for the back, and lying in bed can make the pain worse. It is possible to get the person to become more active again if they understand that their back pain is not life threatening and that moving around will not cause them spinal problems or the pain gets worse. In the same way we can understand emotional pain and anxiety and depression. Techniques can be used to reduce emotional pain. It is helpful to think about or write about our anxieties and depression using language, like writing poetry or the technique of diary writing or journaling. I must say that I have found this a very effective way of helping me to sort out my ideas. With written language, the ideas become translated into concrete words, and we can address them, or at least externalise them. I have kept a journal throughout most of the last year, and some extracts and excerpts from it are featured later on in this book. Poetry is a very moving way of dealing with our emotional hurt, and again, I went through a phase of about 2 months where I wrote poetry about my mental health experiences. I had been composing the words in my head for months, and then it came to me that I needed to write them down, and my poetry just evolved. I called my poems 'Poems for Mental Health'. Again, I have always found music a useful therapy in itself, sitting listening to music can help me relax and also energies me if it is a fast moving track. I would sit for hours listening to Elton John's 'Recover Your Soul' because I found the words so meaningful, or lie on my bed with Classic FM playing whilst I tried to calm my nerves, and get my head into some sort of order. It is a well known therapy tool and I made full use of my music.

I think it is important to stress that I still felt anxiety when I was on the prescribed drug Prozac, and also had feelings of agitation. Sometimes these were worse than others, and I believed that it was my condition. But I find now on Efexor XL that these feelings have gone, and I can now relax knowing that I am not agitated or anxious as a matter of course. Occasionally, when I am doing something new or there is a particularly stressful situation to deal with, then I may feel anxious, but I regard that as normal behaviour and not something to worry about. So, I am pleased to rely on my current prescription for alleviation of this symptom.

Chapter 16 - Depression

Bipolar Affective Disorder used to be known as Manic Depression and still many people like to use the old name. In some ways the term manic depression conjures up the feeling of the illness very well, including mania and depression, so I think it is a very apt name. Bipolar Affective Disorder is a mood disorder, so it is a state of being. All I can say is that I have found the depression states of my condition exceedingly difficult to deal with. One of the worst effects of depression is the difficulty with getting up in the morning. Sometimes this has been caused by the after-effects of the drugs that are prescribed to beat the condition, and then of course it becomes a way of life of lying in bed, not getting up, because there is no job to go to and no particular purpose to getting up and on in life. There is no motivation there to get out and meet the world. The body tends to learn what it is experiencing, so remaining in bed becomes what the body gets used to. I have had tremendous problems with this. Depression has made me insular, and very inward looking at times. I have sometimes been totally unable to contact friends, and maintain social friendships, so that my life has become quite empty. I have had no energy for doing anything, and totally lost the motivation to even think about what to do. My community psychiatric nurse brought me a tape about depression, and when I was in a deeply depressed state I would lie on the bed, listening to this information about depression, and how the tape kept saying that the feelings would pass. Mine never seemed to pass, they were always low, and I felt quite dispirited. However, I took heart from the actual description of the condition of depression, as being like the physical condition diabetes, which needs to be treated, and is no more the fault of anyone who suffers from it than is depression. Depression has made me very tearful at times, and I have spent hours alone in the house crying, wondering what was going to become of me, unable to settle to anything, and wandering around like a lost soul. Sometimes I have experienced real psychotic symptoms with my depression, and have felt terrified by the delusional states I found myself in. I remember sitting on my bed, crying desperately because I was worried about my daughter, and thought of her as this little girl of 4 years old being chased by a fierce Alsatian dog, and how there was nothing that I could do to rescue her. Sometimes I linked my thoughts in with what was on the television, and I imagined that the TV was talking directly to me. Sometimes this could be really unnerving. My husband explained to me that in a time of heightened sensitivity we are very alert as to what information we hear and see, and so of course it may well feel that the TV and radio are talking to us especially. In a depressed state, our senses are very often quite acute, because our bodies need to be able to protect us I expect, so when the balance of our systems is out of kilter, then our senses step in and seem heightened too. This is at one extreme, because at the other, is when our senses seem totally down, and we just sit for hours in a very depressed state, really unable to move or do anything at all. I have been there too. Anti-depressants are prescribed for depression and it is a question of finding the right drug which will make a difference, and help lift our depression. That does not mean to say that we will forever be on prescription drugs, but maybe for a time that is part of the answer. Psychiatrists of ten say that it is a chemical imbalance which causes our condition, and so maybe we need chemicals to provide that balance to our life again. I am not a great believer in a pill for every ill, so it came as quite a shock to me to learn that I would probably have to be on prescribed drugs to improve my mental health for the rest of my life.

Another very useful way to help us with depression is to consider the various complementary therapies. I have tried aromatherapy, which is a thorough massage, using various different oils. I remember on a couple of occasions, I could hardly drag myself along to the health centre, but I was determined to get there, to have a massage. I remember my body felt thoroughly heavy and totally uncoordinated, and my mind was either spinning or just totally lethargic. With aromatherapy you get to lie on a couch for nearly an hour and have this wonderful massage all over your body with various scented oils. The aromatherapist will choose the most appropriate oils for you, depending on how you are feeling, and will carefully blend a mixture together for your skin. The action of massage on your physical body – the arms and the legs and the torso – helps to make you feel in touch with your physical body and along with the scents which reach you, percolate through to your mind, helping to relieve tension and encourage a feeling of peace. I would thoroughly recommend an aromatherapy or massage for those of us suffering from depression. Other ways of paying attention to the body are also helpful in getting the body and mind to fit together. Reiki is an Indian head massage, a gentle treatment, and reflexology is a foot massage, which helps to relax you too. I have tried these and also a pedicure and a manicure when I wished to feel a little spoilt and felt in need of a bit of extra attention to my body. Of course when we are well it is often just as easy to do your own nails, but when you are suffering from depression, it is an effort to do anything, and I for one would certainly not have managed to even cut my nails let alone massage the foot and then paint the toenails. It all made me feel better about myself, which is an important lift when you have depression. Also if you have a good friend who will do this for you I am sure it serves the same purpose.

I think one of the main problems with depression is that we lose our zest for living and getting out there into the market place to interact with people. I always admire those individuals who can get on with their lives, meeting new people and be able to say and do the right kind of things to make their interactions come alive. I have always found that I am on the passive side, and I suppose that is why when I became ill, I have more easily descended into depression. However, that is also why I started on the self-confidence and esteem class, to learn how to be more assertive and I undertook a 10 week course where we learned and re-learned various skills and techniques to help us to get out there. One of them was how to talk to people, and we had practice exercises of moving round the room starting up conversations on safe topics like the weather, did you see the programme on TV last night, have you heard the news about, etc. It was reassuring to me to find that I was actually quite good with a lot of these kinds of interactions, but perhaps I didn't have that much to say about them, because with my depression I was not reading the papers, and did not really keep up with the news, and sometimes I had been totally unable to even watch TV, when my concentration would not let me. It is the same with reading a paper, unless we have concentration, the information can go in one eye and not even reach the brain. If we panic and become anxious about a conversation, then the words the other person says may just go in one ear and not reach the brain either. The people may even become blurs and we may not be truly aware of who it is standing in front of us. We tend to panic and the words and faces just spin around our head. However another useful technique I learned was to take a deep breath and feel calm before entering a room of people, and having the mental calmness to be able to face a conversation with people. After quite a lot of practice in this way I now find it much easier to do – in fact sometimes I actually relish the thought of meeting some new people, and wonder what I will be saying. I find that after the conversation gets going, then it becomes a great deal easier, and I can then forget about me and my worries about myself and what other people think of me, and I can just get on with the conversation and the interaction. It is this worry, and anxiety which comes from depression and not feeling interesting enough for other people to want to talk to, that causes the problem in the first place. So an assertion and self-confidence class is probably a useful tool too.

Another difficult thing about depression is that it makes us feel very lethargic, and we tend to just want to sit around, sometimes it is the effect of the medication which tends to make us very drowsy. So, although people keep saying take some exercise or go to the gym, or make an effort to go swimming, sometimes it is all we can do to get up in the morning and just sit. It may be difficult to go to the shops and select good food, and we may not be up to cooking low fat, high fibre meals to keep us healthy. Instead, we may prefer to comfort eat, on cakes and biscuits or buy ready made food dishes, which are fairly high in sugar and additives. Again, it is difficult when suffering from depression to make an effort with our clothing. Our personal habits may slide, like taking a shower or washing thoroughly each day before dressing. This lack of interest in our appearance does nothing to encourage us to want to go out and meet people, and equally it does nothing to encourage others to want to make the effort to talk to us if the going is tough. I remember well being totally disinterested in what I was going to wear, let alone how my house looked. I had no interest in housework for a long time, and in the end I have been lucky enough to find paid help to do a basic two hour clean for me. This makes the world of difference to me, because I can keep the house looking and feeling clean and tidy and with some of the work being done, there is less for me to cope with. It also means that other family members who may have full and busy lives do not feel burdened with the pressure to start cleaning and tidying your house or even just a room. I now find that it helps to work out the day before if I am going to try and do a particular task like tackling a room which needs a good tidy. This minimal forward preparation helps me feel I am ahead of the game, which is a good way to be. However, when I was in the severest of depressed states, there was no way I could plan ahead, it was hard enough just to exist on a day to day basis, and it was irrelevant, the way I looked or the way my house looked.

With depression, it has always been important for me to have some help and support in a personal sense. For me I have been lucky to have a husband who has tried to give me the necessary care and attention when I needed it. He has also been able to discuss my depression with me and made the time to do this when I wanted to talk about myself and how the illness was affecting my ability to do the housework or to go for a walk, or not to work and perhaps to seem to be losing my friends. However, it is tough on one person to be that all caring support and it is often useful to have some professional support coming into the household to be the listening ear. For months I had a community psychiatric nurse who would call and see me before I was able to make an appointment at the out-patient hospital. This was a useful support for me. However, when I was quite ill at times and almost confined to the house because I was scared to go out and about much, I would have liked a voluntary visitor coming round to see me at least once a week just to talk to me and share a cup of tea and find out how I was. I tended to be quite isolated at home if I was not able to make the effort to go out. For those people who live alone it is particularly important to have help coming into the house if you feel unable to go out and do your shopping, or even to take a little walk in the park on your own, unless you have a strong support network of friends, who will take it in turns to come and help.

To conclude on depression I think that the effects of this condition are exacerbated with time. At first we struggle hard to hang on to that persona and the way of life we have. Through time this gradually becomes eroded. It is not that we decide we do not want that life any more; it is rather that we somehow cannot hold on to it. I have struggled for years trying to recapture that way of life I had where I was up with the lark and about my daily business and looking after the children, and running a busy household. Now, to some extent the pressure is relieved because my children are older and no longer needing the constant attention and care which I would lavish on them. But this has left me with a void in my life, and now I do not need to struggle in the same way. Because I was not out there in the market place at this time of transition in my life, I have been sidelined in the general run of things and find I cannot summon up enthusiasm for developing other areas of my life. No one is out there searching for me, except my family, who still need me and want me, but I mean no other outside agencies are really calling out to me. This has led me to be completely non-assertive in my life style, and I mix in a very small circle. This tends to reinforce the loneliness and isolation and so the depression never seems to go away. Depression seems to be a condition which eats away at your very soul. Over the years it gains more hold over your body and mind, and many aspects of your life are controlled by this condition. The chemical treatments hold the real effects of the chemical imbalance that is depression at bay, but your soul is gradually eaten away and eroded. It takes real determination to hold on to your 'self' to prevent destruction of the personality. A caring and supportive family is the greatest support.

Chapter 17 - Mania

In some ways mania is quite a difficult state to describe because I think it is impossible to realise you are in a manic state until you have been told by the doctors that you suffer from mania and with time you have sufficient insight to understand what that mania is. I did not believe I was suffering from mania at all, at the various times when I became hypo. Looking back now, I can understand my mania, and what it was, but that is only because I now know that I am suffering from bipolar affective disorder and have experienced attacks of mania. I think it is a time of mind expansion and can be quite an exhilarating feeling in a way, although sometimes quite frightening. Sometimes I have felt that I could do anything and become a most important highly paid official in one of the top jobs. I remember sending off job application forms for some highly paid posts, and ringing up for details of others, when I believed they were all within my grasp. I also remember going for a walk with my parents in law and we were visiting an aquarium. I loved seeing the little fish swimming around in their tanks and became quite obsessed with two little fish that were having a game of hide and seek. I believed these fish were my children and I wanted to buy them and take them home. I did not become distressed when I was told the fish were happy there, and that we would not be buying them, so on another level I must have been quite clear that they were not my children! Until earlier this year, when I was put onto a regular dose of Risperdal I have for the last 6 or so years, often experienced my mind wandering as I put it. I thought this was just a normal thing to feel for those of us who are depressed and on anti-depressants. I would be trying to concentrate on something, say a conversation and sometimes my mind would just take off into its own little world, which would possibly be something to do with the conversation or just as likely an extension in my own mind of other connections which I had made. It is not surprising that I found it therefore very difficult to concentrate on where I was and what had to be done next. It is only since I have been taking this Risperdal that I realise it has stopped this regular mind wandering feeling. I now feel my concentration is much better, and I can apply my mind to the task at hand. Again, I feel it is a lot better too since I have started on the anxiety reducing anti-depressant drug Efexor. The combination seems to enable me to concentrate better.

When I was first taken ill, one of the things that happened was that for about three nights I woke up in the night and had to get up and wanted to be very busy. I wanted to sort out photographs, and I wanted to write letters to my children, and I wanted to make sure that everything would be in order should I die, because I thought that I was perhaps going to die that night. I remember getting on my dressing gown, putting on the lights and sitting in the study working away. My husband did not know what to make of this, and all he could do was tell me to go back to bed and that I could do all these things in the morning. Luckily I did eventually go back to bed as he had requested, but that was the start of my mania as I put it. I think mania is a type of hyper-excitability and it is quite a powerful sort of a chemical reaction in the body which seems to give us excess energy and ideas without tiredness. It also seemed to be a step into a more extraordinary world which I normally did not frequent.

For example, on one occasion I was going for a walk in Richmond Park with my husband when I suddenly got the feeling that my husband was taking me to my death. I was not afraid because he was there with me, but I thought I was Anne Boleyn, and was on my way to have my head chopped off. I remember we were walking along a long, windy path through the park and I kept wanting to know where we were going. It was quite unnerving and the feelings were very strong. Another time I was in Wales with my husband and my son, and we were visiting one of their lovely castles. There was a sign displayed about the history of the castle at the entrance to the buildings, and we read this before going in. As we walked around the place I had the strangest feeling that I was back there in the times of the life of the castle about 200 years before, and that I was a part of the scene then. I had a strange feeling of drifting around the place, and I did not want to leave the ruins, because I so enjoyed my time there. I also felt very tired immediately after that and quite disorientated as to where I was being taken in the car by my husband. Another time I experienced mania was when I believed I was a James Bond girl in one of his films and I was being driven in a car by my husband to Liverpool – but really it was a movie. Another character in the movie was Osama Bin Laden and I believed that somehow I was harbouring him, in the same sort of way as a mother would look after her son. But it was rather terrifying. I described it to the psychiatrist as different thoughts, that one minute I thought one thing and then I was turned around and thought something else. I asked him if he knew what I meant, and he seemed to understand that how I was describing my life on the move.

After I had recovered from the first bout of my illness in the late 90's I started doing a management course at Westminster University, in their business school – a very intensive post-graduate level course for women going into management. I really enjoyed it and worked exceedingly hard. Sometimes when I overextended myself I felt my mind starting to wander and it became too difficult to concentrate, but on the whole, after a rest or a change of scene I managed well. Towards the end when there was the pressure of writing the essays and getting our presentation ready I felt my mania in the sense that I found the excess energy to work exceptionally hard to get the work all done on time – once staying up until 2 in the morning to finish the written work for our team presentation and then carrying on as normal the next morning. It was a very productive time. However, when the course had finished and I was at home again, there was the extreme tiredness to deal with and I felt exhausted for about 3 months. After recovery, during which I basically spent time sitting around, resting, I started to feel well enough to get my thoughts together to apply for a good job. I landed quite a good job, and applied myself to working there in a fairly senior position, at management level. However, I had a very bad experience in this job, where I felt badly treated by my employers, but unable to make satisfactory changes in the working day to improve my position. I was on Prozac all this time, but was not currently being treated by the psychiatrist. This was before any diagnosis of manic depression, and it was just thought that I suffered from depression. So frequently my mind would wander, and I would work with excess energy at a great pace. I do not think my employers appreciated my obvious talents, and unfortunately this did not lead to a good working relationship with them. However, I am inclined to think that they would have had trouble with anyone, and therefore I do not believe my illness led me to losing the job. However, when the employment came to an end, this left me with a very bad impression of working life, and it set me into a downward spiral for quite some time, leading me to see the psychiatrist again.

Eventually I tried a little bit of secretarial work, as in fact I had been an experienced secretary in my own business. Again, I found that too much, I think because my medication was too heavy and I always felt tired and my head used to spin, so I gave up on employment for another full year and remained quietly at home, trying to recover. During most of this last year, I was under the psychiatrist and we have gradually got round to finding the best medication for me with my new diagnosis of manic depression. It seems to have worked. But there have been long years of peaks and troughs, and ups and downs, and although I have tried my best to work I was just totally unable to take on a new job, albeit even a fairly straightforward one. I wondered really how an employer would take to finding out an employee had manic depression, especially when I did not feel able to cope. However, I did start doing some regular voluntary work after a really bad episode of mania and I have gradually built up from those two days a week, to being able a year later to take on a part-time paid post. It is small steps little by little, which enabled me to gradually build up my self esteem again. It is amazing how my self confidence became totally shattered with the bad experience of work in the interim years, followed by a diagnosis of manic depression, and the knowledge that I would have to be on medication for the rest of my life.

In the summer before I started the 2 days a week voluntary work, I had a really bad manic experience. I felt suicidal. My mind had really disintegrated I feel and kept going off into flights of fancy, and I thought I was no use to anyone or for anything. At the time I was on Risperdal and Prozac and felt completely drugged. I hated it. Each and every day in the summer all I could do was lie out in the sun on a lounger and wait for the day to pass. I could not concentrate to read, and I did not want to listen to music. This was one of the most awful periods of my life. I could not summon any enthusiasm for anything. I could not bear the thought of my life just continuing in this awful way. It was about this time that the psychiatrist suggested I might be better to go into hospital for an assessment and treatment, but I would not. I clung on to what I felt was my identity as Anne, living at home with my husband. I felt if I surrendered to living in a psychiatric unit that I would not know where I was and how to get back to being me. I did not want to go into a psychiatric hospital. I feared that would be the end. But it is a very frightening situation to find yourself lost at home, and in your own mind, and yet not believing there is any hope for the future. Thank God that my husband helped me by phoning me regularly every day just to check on how I was, and he always came back from work for my appointments with the psychiatrist. Somehow I managed to get through this dreadful time and I was taken off Risperdal, remaining on Prozac.

Chapter 18 - A Diagnosis of Manic Depression

Here are the written words which defined my diagnosis. I believe it is traditionally a very difficult condition to diagnose, and takes many years of illness and ineffective treatment to arrive at a diagnosis. Mine is dated 6th September 2002, and says,

"This was her second episode of illness that I think is probably best diagnosed as a mixed affective disorder. This means a form of bipolar affective disorder when people get a mixture of being low and being high at the same time." ... "I have also suggested that she may benefit from a mood stabiliser such as Lithium, again to prevent further episodes. She was quite happy to accept the Prozac but was reluctant to take the Lithium. We therefore agreed she would stay on the Prozac alone for the time being."

Throughout the next year it was a bit of a roller coaster of trying drugs and then relapses, and in the new year I was put back on to Risperidone, an anti-psychotic drug, which I remain on and have been told now that I should take this for the foreseeable future. I also asked about the Prozac which did not seem to have curbed my anxiety, "She has considerably improved although she is still anxious at times." So the psychiatrist suggested I come off the Prozac, as it can make patients feel empty. So for 8 weeks I was only on Resperidone, and enjoyed the way that I seemed to be able to feel again after so many years of anti-depressants. However, after 6 weeks or so when the effects of the Prozac had worn off I became anxious, and agitated in particular, and so, on the next psychiatric appointment my psychiatrist changed the anti-depressant to Efexor XL modified release capsules, which does seem to have curbed my anxiety.

On Risperidone and Efexor XL I now try and live my life but I have put the prescribed drugs on the back burner, and consider my manic depression diagnosis as an aid to treatment, not as a way to live broadcasting that fact. I am relieved that I no longer feel so anxious, and can live with the drugs. However, I still feel depressed and can no longer do all the things which filled my life prior to my breakdown. After a Diet and Lifestyle course organised by the Psychiatric team at the hospital I asked for my Risperidone to be cut in half, because of the effects of weight gain with this anti-psychotic drug. I am managing fine on half the dose and in fact seem to have a bit more energy. I have also been trying hard to lose some weight which has made me feel a bit more confident in my own ability to determine my own care and future. After all I am a partner in the process, an active partner, and the services exist for people like me, not on their own. However, it is taking a considerable effort on my part to make this effort, and it is easy to get lost again, in the general mire of troubles.

Chapter 19 - Fighting Against the Medical Establishment

I am pleased that I have a medical diagnosis because it assists in my treatment by the medical profession and it also helps me to find out a bit more about my medical condition. Since diagnosis I have been able to pick up different books which give accounts, either as medical authorities or case study stories, and patients' experiences, like this book aims to be. However I do not want to remain now just as a manic depressive. I am still me, and I happen to be suffering from manic depression, but I also have a family, and two children, and a husband and a few friends, and I aim to get back into work and develop my friendship circle. Now that I know it seems easier. It took a while for it to sink in because I did not want and still do not want to be ill. For me, any opportunity to cut down the prescribed drugs is a good idea. I used to be embarrassed that I had a mental health difficulty and saw a psychiatrist, but now I accept it, even though I know that some others have called me 'nutter' and 'loony'.

I think it is a question of getting everything in perspective. A medical diagnosis is useful, in one sense but there are various alternative treatments and a holistic approach to life which militates against emphasising this medical model. However, I cannot get away from the very real fact that I am on prescribed medication and that to date I have not found anything else which gives me some satisfaction or positive approach to living life. I can only hope that a book like this will reach psychiatrists and enable them to understand something of the thinking and feelings behind the patient with manic depression. It is just as it is – not overstated and I hope not underdone.

I have though read quite a bit of the more campaigning and radical models of mental health treatment. I feel it is important to involve the patient in patient care, and state that it is vital to listen to what patients have to say. At the point of crisis though, it is the medical profession which can hold the key to treatment, based on the previous experiences of earlier patients. It is vital to work in partnership with the family too. That is why each patient does have that key responsibility to give back some of their feelings and experiences on treatment to the medical profession to enable practitioners to improve and perfect their care.

Chapter 20 - Alternatives as a Supplement to Traditional Medicine

In my early twenties I did four or five years of yoga and so knew about its beneficial effects. For the last three years my husband and I have been members of a health club and go to regular weekly sessions of yoga and swimming. I have also more recently started attending Body Balance, which is a choreographed exercise class originating I believe from New Zealand, and uses postures and movements from yoga, tai chi, and Pilates. When we first enrolled in the class I discussed with the teacher my mental health needs and my depression and I was told that this is a very good class for me. It certainly is very gentle exercise but it really gets you moving, and I do feel that it has loosened me up and helped me to become more flexible in a way that yoga alone cannot do. I have followed a self confidence class and tried to enrol on a NLP, neuro-linguistic programming course, of positive thinking, but it was full up. To treat myself and try and reward myself for good progress, I have had some aromatherapy, reflexology and even a Reiki session at a complementary therapy taster session. The psychiatric outpatient clinic provided the course on diet and lifestyle and my pharmacist suggested that in addition to the anti-depressant and anti-psychotic the only other useful pill might be a multi-vitamin, although my psychiatrist says that if I am following a good diet then this is not necessary. Care of self is important when depression weighs down on our shoulders, so again I treated myself to a pedicure now and again – when I was really depressed and lethargic it was more than I could do to even bend towards my toenails. Journaling, as writing therapy, art and music therapy have also been useful tools in the fight against depression. I have also over the years tried to develop a really balanced life in terms of home and work. By work, I mean things I get involved in outside the home, which in my case has been mainly voluntary work, but recently again, I have been attempting to procure paid work too. CBT – cognitive behavioural therapy is something my daughter is a great believer in, and as a technique for identifying my needs and behaviour she suggested to me that I take up journaling and handed me my first small book to write in. She told me about CBT and I then could ask the psychiatrist about it. He said I did not need it, but yet I know people who see the psychologist for this kind of help on referral from the psychiatrist. However, when I reviewed my journals for this book I saw to some extent that I had made progress in my diaries by working through a lot of my feelings by reading books and then taking notes about the points which I felt were very pertinent. I suppose it was my form of cognitive behavioural therapy. It has certainly made me aware of my feelings of unresolved grief and loss. Anti-depressants work to release serotonin in the brain and I believe it is the amyglada which is responsible for the release of this chemical there. The fear response also starts in the amyglada as I recently understood from a TV programme, and so perhaps my brain has got rather mixed up with its responses to fear and pleasure because of a previous overload when I had so many different pressures all pressing in on me. The fight or flight response to threats of danger is well known and perhaps my body just had one too many threats of danger to deal with before it decided to go into flight response. Whatever the cause of my depression and bipolar affective disorder I am pleased that I have tried so many alternatives and self-help therapies to supplement the traditional approach of prescribed medication. Unfortunately though I have not found a cure, I only wish I could.

Perhaps manic depression is another name for post traumatic stress disorder and so those of us with bipolar affective disorder seem to have so much in common with e.g. soldiers suffering after war. There was quite an active campaign, which I supported, for those soldiers from the First World War whose families and friends were campaigning to pardon them from the cowardice with which they had been labelled. These soldiers were those men who were 'shot at dawn' for cowardice in the field of battle, after various stories of battle fear. I believe that these men were suffering from stress – in other words post traumatic stress disorder – after fighting on the front line, and taking more than they could take, they felt they could take no more fighting. Instead of being treated with compassion they were treated as though they had cold bloodedly decided to run away from the battle. These soldiers, I believe there were 309 of them, were then shot at dawn. No treatment for their condition was provided in those days, and they were shot. Because of my condition I felt great compassion for them and took to writing letters to my MP about the campaign in support of these maltreated soldiers. I have also been reading quite a lot about people who were compulsorily given ECT treatment and have suffered appalling memory loss on top of their depression and stress. We still have a lot to learn about mental health and the consequent problems of mental illness. There have to be alternatives to these inhumane and degrading treatments.

Chapter 21 - How My Family Coped

They always say it is harder for the family to cope, than for the person afflicted with the condition to deal with their illness. I don't know. So far it is only me who has been ill in this round of manic depression. I know my family has found it tough too. My daughter at 15, according to my husband, asked around her friends to see what their experiences of mental health problems with mothers was. It was not good. To some extent I think my son alternated between ignoring the situation and pretending it was not happening, to speaking to me directly saying things like mad mothers, and mental health loonies, repeating words and phrases he has heard, so I think he has been in a quandary, and I cannot seem to help him with that, except by trying to live my life and get better. My husband has been the saving face and the strong arm behind the family in this stressful time. Prior to my illness it was always me who fixed the appointments for this and that, and dealt with all the arrangements in relation to care of the children. This all changed on my breakdown, and I felt quite left out at first. My husband David has gradually become the carer, and you can read my poem about this later in the book.

David was a journalist in Guildford when I met him first. I was a social worker. We clicked and both seemed to have the need for sharing in our life together. We both had problems, but we focussed on the positive things we could do together. We got involved in campaigning work, we went on marches, he was active in the union, and I was involved with pressure groups.

We both wanted to change the world, and so we hoped to do that together. I think we worked hard at that philosophy over the years and we have managed with others to make some changes.

Same with our problems. We have tried together to combat my depression, and David has never ceased to accompany me on psychiatrist's appointments, or to talk to me about my feelings of depression. He has also been the one to take me to the Doctor throughout the years when I needed that medical intervention. We do not know what else we can do. We read books, we listen to the radio programmes, we talk to people, and I get involved with mental health issues when I can. We went to our local MIND AGM this year, all in an effort to get up to speed with the world of mental health. What else can we do?

My children have shared with me their thoughts about my illness and when I have triumphed they have rejoiced with us. They never cease to encourage me to make progress, and to climb out of the pit of isolating depression. With my family around about me I have also tried to improve my condition because I know that they all care about me. With them, my suicidal thoughts have never been active ones, just because I have all the love of a family round about me. My mother in law tells me that when she first came down to help all those years ago when I had a breakdown, she could just feel the love, and she says that she explained this to my daughter who naturally at 14 was most concerned and worried about her mother. When you have love you can conquer fear.

Chapter 22 - Poems for Mental Health

Earlier in 2003 I felt in quite a creative mood, but at the same time pretty depressed about the long lasting nature of my illness. I felt it would be quite helpful for me to write some poems and after a brief time of thinking about what exactly to write I quickly wrote a short collection. They were descriptive, non rhyming blank verse, and I felt quite proud of my achievement, as they covered a wide range of my feelings in yet quite a different way. So, what to do with them. I sent them all to my psychiatrist by email. I could not print them out as my printer was broken, so the only thing I could do with them was email them to the doctor. I sent him a message saying I had written these poems as a way of trying to understand my feelings throughout my illness and of the progress which I had made. On the following psychiatric appointment he said he had received my poems and printed them out and kept a copy at the front of my file. He said he had been moved by them and intended to share them with his team at the Nelson Hospital. Here is the collection of my Poems for Mental Health.

Poems for Mental Health by Anne Brocklesby

Diagnosis and Self Diagnosis

Self-diagnosis is a dangerous condition.
I know because I have tried it once for a very long time.
It isn't that I wanted to be a doctor, or anything medical.
In fact, I am a traditionalist in the sense of believing that doctors are in charge.
However, I like to know what is wrong with me, when it is wrong with me, and to take a positive role in the process.
I used to think it was just depression as did my doctor.
I used to have strange feelings in my head where I imagined fancifully.
I would think that my children were little fish, peeping out from behind a rock to dart in and out of sight.
I wanted to buy those little fish at the aquarium and take them home.
I was checked in this behaviour by my relatives who explained about the little creatures
Being happy in situ, and that I would have needed a fish tank to cope with them.
So, family are important in the diagnostic and self diagnosis procedure.
We must listen to others or we are in danger of losing touch with reality.

Language and thoughts are external.

So, today in the post I received a letter from my psychiatrist.

It is a copy of the one he writes to my GP.

It says, "I saw this lady on 22nd April 2003. She is well in herself and her mood is stable.

She complains of feeling lethargic and an inner feeling of emptiness.

We had a long discussion about her medications.

I suggested that it is important that she remain on the Risperidone, but the Prozac is less important. It is the Prozac that may be contributing to the feeling of emptiness which she described and finds distressing.

We therefore agreed that she may remain on the Risperidone at a dose of 4mg a day, but that she discontinues the Prozac."

The psychiatrist emphasises the importance of remaining on the Risperidone in order to prevent further relapses. He has arranged to see me again in 8 weeks time.

This joint approach to diagnosis and treatment is helpful. It makes me feel that I am in charge of my own future too.

I like getting copy letters about my care – it is important to me and for my self-esteem.

Also, I find it useful now that I have a diagnosis of bipolar affective disorder, to read about this condition.

I bought two books – one written by a doctor for patients and their families with manic depression,

And the other being a collaborative approach by an actress with bipolar affective disorder, and a medical specialist in the field.

They both give me more information which is an important part of management of the condition.

In reading these books I can identify with some of the feelings and situations explored in the book, and this helps me recognise that I am not alone.

Also, now that I have a diagnosis, I have the option of joining a self-help group.

In my view it opens the door to further progress, rather than just labelling me.

So, I have a particular condition, but I am also me, that unique, special human being.

And my family value me in their own particular way, and together with other support contacts and friends, help me value myself and start looking to the future.

Sleuthing

It's an amazing feat – I now have a diagnosis.
And I believe it to be correct. I'm reading a book about it to be sure
Because I feel I need to know too
That this is the way I need to be treated.
But it's taken a long, long time. Is it 18 years?
After years and years of sorrow and tears.
The medical profession has taken me into their confidence
And tried to explain my condition.
It is bipolar affective disorder – formerly called manic depression.
A long time ago I read a book about post-natal depression
I remember I felt as though I might be suffering from that at the time.
I also read a lot about hyperactivity in children, though thinking now
It would have been better to read about hypersensitivity.
I sleuthed over the years to try and discover more about these feelings.
I occasionally saw a doctor usually about gynaecological things.
Then, seven years ago I had what I call a nervous breakdown.
It followed some personal stress, but developed into unexpected mania.
I was treated for depression with various drugs, like Valium, and risperdal and Prozac and remained on the latter one for nearly 7 years

With a couple of breaks where I tried to wean
myself off drugs.
It did not work for me; I became ill again and now
am on risperdal.
What I understand now is that I am feeling better
and able to write poetry.
My words are better because I can concentrate. I
am getting better.
Psychiatry is a success story, so I am relieved.
So is my doctor, that I can get better, being on
medication.
I have not quite got used to it yet, but I'm trying.
It's far better that I learn to live again a productive
life
To increase my voluntary work to the point where I
trust myself
And feel confident enough to seek a paid job.
This task is one 'to do'.
What progress from 8 months ago where I was just
trying 'to be'?
I was desperate and did not know which way to
turn, so I was invited
Along to a support group in the church.
Once a week I had my own group meeting where we
prayed together.
I had just had a diagnosis and I felt lost.
Now 3 seasons further on, I have also moved on.
I am learning to be at peace with myself, and return
to
A healthy, balanced life. At least I know now.
So I'm hoping to meet plenty of other people, and
talk to them too.
Bit by bit about my experiences.

Sleuthing is hard work. There's a lot more to do.

_____

Unceremoniously Dumped

It was when I was vulnerable and feeling lost.
No one seemed to be helping me professionally.
I had appointments, then I was left alone.
I no longer saw the psychiatrist and was referred
back to my GP.
I had said I wanted to try and get a job.
Now I think that was totally unrealistic.
10 months further on, and I'm still not confident
enough
To job search, let alone hold down paid work.
So, somehow I managed to have an appointment
with someone new.
I had been referred to the Occupational Therapist.
I remember waiting day by day for the
appointment.
In between times I was at home, resting, feeling
tired and depressed.
So I pinned a lot of hope on this appointment.
I had recently been diagnosed as manic depressive
But it had not sunk in.
I felt tired and lethargic, but I was not mentally ill.
I even came off Risperdal and I felt a wreck.
I had no confidence. I cried so easily.
I felt very sensitive and vulnerable, but I did not feel
ill.
The day of my appointment arrived and I went to
see the OT.

I walked along – 20 minutes to the hospital – it felt like an hour.
I was tired when I got there, and agitated, and after introducing myself to her I cried.
It was so exhausting being ill and short of words.
Nothing made sense.
Why was I there?
Surely I could get a job without specialist help? But no – I couldn't.
I remember how I desperately wanted to appear normal.
But it was all too much for me and I cried and felt so sad.
Why was I sitting opposite an OT? And talking about myself?
At least I wasn't talking to myself then.
I agreed to do some voluntary work to get myself on my feet again,
And arranged to go with the OT to the volunteer bureau –
She would make another appointment for us.
So, some 2-3 weeks later she came to my house and took me along for the appointment.
I wouldn't have made it without her, but she thought I seemed fine.
I put on a brave face at first, but then again I cried.
As I was introduced to the volunteer bureau, that was my only dealings with the OT.
So again I was dumped, unceremoniously, to get on with life on my own.
There never was anyone to talk to.

There Never Is Anyone To Really Speak To

Oh help – I need someone to talk to.
Someone who will listen to me, maybe come for a
coffee
Or talk to me slowly about their life too.
Why is there no one there?
I thought there was care in the community?
But there's no care for me – there's no one to talk
to.
I need someone to be there for me, just for me, now
or when I feel lonely.
It feels as though I am alone – deserted on this
planet.
The last one left alive here, but what a lonely life!
There's no one to talk to.
There's no one to speak with.
Everyone is busy with their own life, and talking
away
On the phone, in the street in the shops, on the radio
and TV
But there's no one for me.
No one is here where I am, alone, feeling lonely but
Unable to really speak up for myself.
I feel lost and withdrawn but want someone to speak
to.
I once tried the Samaritans, but it's a bit anonymous
over the phone.
I want to see someone and talk to them.

I'd really like to have a voluntary visitor, someone who would come to my house and see me and talk to me.

I tried to get a voluntary visitor, and phoned an agency, who sent round volunteers, but you needed to qualify for their service, and I didn't so I couldn't have a voluntary visitor.

I'm not elderly or housebound as such, although I often felt completely trapped in my own house, afraid to go out.

Then I was sometimes too tired to concentrate for the radio and the TV and I couldn't read.

I felt tired, but I would have liked a voluntary visitor – someone to speak to.

There never was anyone to speak to!

Doctor and Patient

Her behaviour was inappropriate was one of the descriptions the Doctor used.

She was paranoid was another.

My psychiatrist writes me copy letters of the reports he regularly sends to my GP about my care.

I'm grateful for these – they provide a link between one appointment and the next, and describe my behaviour.

I find this very useful as an objective test of who I am and the way I have presented to the doctor for attention.

Usually I cannot remember who said what, unless I write about it straight after the interview as I sometimes do.

Last time for example we held a discussion about the effects of my medication, and agreed that I would continue on one drug, as prescribed, which I had been getting used to for some 4 or so months, and the other drug I would stop.

We discussed, or rather he told me and I heard about the side effects which can sometimes make you feel empty and lethargic.

So we decided and I agreed, I would stop that drug. I wanted to feel, and I wanted to try and be me again, not some drugged up patient who can't say boo to a goose.

Sometimes I've ended up saying, 'yes doctor', when I've been given a psychiatric opinion.

I mean I do not know, how can I possibly equal the expertise of a doctor who's studied psychiatry for more years than I've been ill.

I think I know myself, but I need that objective assessment of my condition.

It is a very personal relationship this – telling my doctor how I feel, and how I've been

But it's very difficult to describe my feelings, especially if I'm feeling paranoid, or I'm obsessed about some detail of my childhood.

But I try. I've been feeling empty for 7 years doctor.

Why I wonder do I bring this up now, when I've not mentioned it before?

Is it because the other medication I've been on is starting to work and I now am able to collect my thoughts and describe the concentration of feelings? I think so.

Also, I'm getting to know my psychiatrist now and because the medication is working we seem to have struck a rapport.

He is pleased that I can get better on medication, and I am relieved my thoughts are starting to focus, and to stop wandering around my head.

This reinforces the belief that psychiatry as a model of care can and does work, so we both feel the doctor/patient relationship is worthwhile.

I'm learning through experience to have confidence in my psychiatrist, which is a very important step when we are talking about problems with the mind, which translate to bodily functions.

Let us build on this Doctor and Patient relationship.

Self-Help and Survival

Yes we have a responsibility for our own health, after we have seen our doctor.

The professional opinion is a good starting point for our action.

It grounds us to the medical model. Which we may choose to complement or supplement.

Many doctors nowadays believe in self-help and patient care may well include complementary therapy.

We have moved a long way from the paternalistic view where the professional doctor always knows best.

Many people believe in taking a second opinion and will discuss their care at some length.

The economics of health care are very complicated. As a patient I appreciate the consultant and GP care I have had.

I have been told about various self-help and educational resources to supplement my care.

These include for example, counselling sessions and support health groups.

I have taken a counselling course for about 3 months and found that beneficial in understanding the true position I was in, aside from the medical diagnosis.

It is crucial to really be able to comprehend the all-round situation.

Why is it that I might choose to take this treatment, or follow that course of action?

I need to know what I think about my health and social care.

I need to understand my feelings about my illness, so that I can take up offers of help.

I need to be able to evaluate support groups on offer.

Do I want to meet other people who are in a similar position to me?

Do I want to share my feelings in a support group for people with a similar diagnosis?

All these are crucial factors to find out about.

I want to do more than survive.

Although sometimes that is the scenario – how can I survive?

Life has to be more than existence on a day to day basis.

So, I need to learn to help myself, to find out what else is on offer, and how that might be just what I need.

Not Wanting To Be Institutionalised

I haven't yet been admitted to hospital for mental illness, although my doctor did ask me.

I declined the offer because I did not want to be institutionalised.

I had the freedom of choice.

I did not have to think about it, I just knew.

I did not want to give up on the tenuous hold I had on my life at that time, so I knew it was best to struggle on.

Life at home was fine, because I knew what was what.

I knew my room, and the activities I could get involved in, and I liked that.

It was safe, because it was comforting and comfortable.

So I did not want to go in for observation, or for a rest, I said no.

But many of my friends have been into hospital and some have talked about their experiences.

Yes, for some it was a rest, a security, when they felt unable to cope at home, and it was the right thing to do.

For some they missed the independence, of being able to go for a walk when they wanted to.

For others the hospital setting was the regularity that they needed.

It gave the doctors and nurses, their carers, the time to sort out a change in medication, and see how they were coping with this alteration.

It meant that the user could be closely observed by the carers, and hopefully therefore get the care he or she needed.

There is always the danger though that the strength of the carers around you makes you feel safe in itself, so you want to stay on.

It is easy to get into a routine at the hospital, with regular meals being provided and the day to day existence of the wards and their visitors.

Perhaps, for some, there comes a point where they feel it is easier on the inside, so they want to stay.

This becomes the danger of institutionalisation, especially if there is a difficulty with medication, and stabilising the care needed.

At what point do we decide that the stigma of hospital admission is worth it, and we decide it is necessary?

Of course, there comes a point if the doctor decides that it is essential, then we really have no choice.

It is at this point that the issue of institutionalisation does not really come into the picture at all, because we need the essential care.

So, stigma and institutionalisation are not relevant at the point of admission, it is just later, when we are getting better that it matters.

Then, that age old problem of society's definition of mental illness comes into play.

Society thinks that if you have a mental illness you are dangerous and need to be inside.

Then, once inside you are labelled with the definition of institutionalised care.

So, really, as yet we cannot win, until we decide to talk about our experiences.

We need to speak up and say that mental illness is treatable, and that mental health is the aim.

We may be institutionalised or not,

We may be able to cope with care in the community.

It's just that we do not want to be stigmatized by society. That's all.

Loneliness and Despair

Loneliness is a three syllable word, but it sounds so sad.

We need to remember the music which goes with the sounds, so we don't feel so bad.

Good lyrics, rhyme and songs always have the power to cheer us up.

And everything is imbued with meaning when we have rare, exposed emotions.

We understand that the words really speak to us.
It's like listening to the radio or television
We are finely attuned to the meanings of words and phrases
It's like we really understand the meaning of meanings.
Our heightened awareness carries us through.
Have you ever felt that the words are just for you?
I have, and it's quite a powerful medium.
Imagine getting your message across to someone who is really listening for inspiration.
It's vital to appreciate the feelings of loneliness before you try and get through to us.
It doesn't just mean there's no one to talk to – it's a whole lot more.
It's much deeper, and describes an emptiness of the wound and the soul within.
It means this is a wake-up call for us all.
We need to understand what it's like to feel lonely.
Imagine that suddenly all your previous life experiences do not count and that you are thrown in at the deep end
To see if you sink or swim.
Now that is loneliness.
Imagine that your previous confidantes and friends no longer seem to comprehend what you are saying.
That you are still speaking up and saying what you think but that your words seem to fall on deaf ears.
I suppose it's a bit like paranoia – aloneness.
Imagine being suddenly alone, not with the luxury of a lovely desert island with palm trees and gently lapping waves,

But say in a dark, damp cave, where the occasional screech of a bat or the batting of wings can be heard, but not seen.

Then, imagine being trapped at the bottom of a deep well, and unable to see anything, or climb up or out of the pit.

Then add time.

And it seems like an endless nothingness.

Now perhaps that is loneliness, but it is very difficult if not impossible to put into words.

What happens next?

There may be people anxiously peering down that well trying to help and straining to see something, but not able to make any actual contact whatever.

There may be an exit to the cave, just round the next corner, but you don't know that, and there's no light.

So, there's help round the bend or above the deep cavern, but no way to access it, and we don't know it's there.

Gosh – now that's isolation and loneliness.

Imagine the feelings of loneliness and how that would lead to wondering if you'd ever get out of there ever?

So, is that despair? I think it is.

It's a wonder that we manage to survive despair, but we do.

My Carer

Let me tell you about my carer. He is a man named David.
He is my husband of 25 years, and friend for 5 years before that.
My carer cares for me by loving me in a tough kind of way.
Not for him the gentle easing, rather the necessary push and pull.
Because I am not an easy person to care for.
I demand attention. I need to be cared for.
But it was not always this way and maybe won't always be the same.
I don't know. I hope not.
But for 7 years I have been looked after with care and love.
Before that I felt as though I was the carer, for my husband and 2 children – a full time job.
My life centred round providing for their care.
Until I became ill with a multitude of pressures.
Then I became the cared for, the one who was looked after.
And I have needed that care. He looks after me.
Sometimes we go for a walk and he will encourage me on.
Or to a yoga class and he will say let's go.
Every time I complete a task I feel better.
He also can feel success at my achievement.

Just like a parent is happy at the child's reward, for completing a lesson.
He is my teacher, helping me to learn again how to do it.
It may be a walk or a process of pruning the plants in the garden.
Or getting up instead of 729 reasons just to stay in bed.
He is here for me to help me and he makes my day.
So day by day we learn together.

There's still A Lot of Hope

Day by day I've lived for quite a long time.
It's helped me survive in this dreadful mix of coming and going.
Not knowing how I would feel when I woke in the morning, or what would be happening during the day either.
Somehow we have managed to get through another year.
Before I was ill I used to get up regularly at the appointed time and carry out a day's work, whether it be in the house, or in the office.
Each day was part of a pattern, not an isolated incident to be dealt with.
Somehow I was robbed of that security when manic depression struck.
All I knew was that I did not feel able to control my life or what was going on around me.

It would be a question of staggering, trying to do what I knew had to be done.

I would attempt to get on the washing in the machine, and then go to get some shopping. My day was limited by these basics.

In between times, I felt so tired, and I had to retire to my bed to rest.

I got to think an awful lot about myself and why I was there, which probably made it worse.

But I remember struggling through the day with the radio on.

Gentle music of the classical variety was helpful.

I could not understand what they were saying on radio 4, or any kind of discussion programme. I did not want to watch the TV.

If I did turn on the TV either the programme was meaningless to me, or the TV seemed to be talking words of wisdom to me, which happens I hear when you have heightened sensitivity.

Milestones in the day were important, like getting up and having a shower which was an accomplishment in itself, before I even got dressed.

Then spending time existing was important too.

It would be enough for me to even think of picking up a book.

My concentration was hopeless.

I could not read – ANYTHING at all.

I felt so useless, unable to move around, not doing anything.

And by previous and usual standards, seemingly wasting my time,

Just waiting for the day to pass.

Oh those were most tormented times for me and for my family.

Many are the time my husband returned home after a day's work and then set to make the supper for us.

I felt so useless, so unable to cope, so desperate.

I seemed to have lost my friends too, because I had nothing to say, and nothing to talk about, nothing as a bite for conversation.

I had no energy to phone my friends, so would only speak to those who phoned me, and over the years this has diminished.

When I was feeling very low, there seemed to be no one to talk to during the day, no one at all, and I even tried to get a voluntary visitor, but there was no one for me, because I was not elderly or housebound.

I did not qualify for a visitor, so I was alone.

I did because of my religious beliefs make an approach to the church that welcomed me in and invited me to a regular weekly prayer group.

For this group was my lifeline, and even though I felt bad, I made the effort to go to the group every week on a Thursday.

For some time this was all I did on my own.

The group helped me with acceptance for myself, and I responded by really joining the group and for some 8 months I have attended weekly, apart from when I have been taken away on holiday by my husband.

Somehow he always struggled to look after me, despite being in full time work, and having a very busy day which he needed all his energies for in the day time.

We struggled on, and eventually through contact with the occupational therapist, I was introduced to the local volunteer bureau, for voluntary work.
I was on the conveyor belt towards work, firstly by becoming a volunteer, to gain confidence by getting out in the morning to a place of work, and secondly to experience life in the workplace again.
All this takes so much energy, my own personal energy and that of my husband and carer.
I was encouraged every day to get up to the workplace which I started at and am still doing 2 days a week.
At the beginning my medication was not yet stabilised and I found the work quite hard.
I struggled through the computer work, feeling a bit dazed, and unable to see very clearly.
But still I did the work, and struck up acquaintances again in the world of work.
I found it very satisfying to be able to say that I was doing fundraising computer work at Crimestoppers Trust two days a week.
At first, because it exhausted me so much I had to rest when I returned home from the voluntary work, because my energies were depleted.
Gradually over time I have managed to do my day's work there and then return home and still do the shopping and the preparation and cooking for the evening meal.
Now I'm even thinking of trying to get a little paid work.
I have made contact with the Department of Employment's worker who helps people who have a disability get back into the world of work.

I have an appointment set up to go and talk to her, to see if there's any possibility of work for me, on a part time basis.
I'll keep you informed.
So you see, there's still a lot of hope.

Looking Inward

When I'm well there's a spring in my step and I am always interested in what is going on around me.
Now that I'm not well, my thoughts are usually directed inwards.
It seems as though I have to contemplate myself in the deepest recesses
In my brain and my mind to see what is going on and why this is happening.
I need to make that conscious effort to open my eyes and look around.
Looking inward is the strangest feeling.
It is a necessary part of the condition, wherein we inhabit our mind.
And our body seems rather superfluous at that time.
I remember spending hours and hours just thinking, and trying to work out why things were like this.
I seemed to be unconscious of time, and unconscious to what others were thinking.
I needed to spend that time alone in my mind, trying to make connections which were important to me.
How often did I relive those times of my mother's illness and the aloneness I had felt at the time.

Yet I was living in the present, some 30 years on, it was almost like an anniversary, but what had brought it on?

My mother had died the day after I graduated from university, after a long illness bravely dealt with. So, one of the most exciting days in your life – your graduation – for me was completely abhorrent, I hated it, and I will never forget the feeling of impending doom.

Yet the next day, after my mother had died, I felt some relief that she was free from suffering, and to some extent joyous, because I had grieved my mother in those long years leading up to her death. So, really my emotions were completely back to front, the wrong emotions being displayed for inappropriate reasons.

This was the result of all the years of torment.

As the oldest daughter I suppose I just learned to grin and bear it, I mean just what else did you do in those days.

Nowadays, there are services for children like me, called young carers support worker.

As it was, I had no one to talk to about my worries and my problems when I was a teenager, and I felt alone, so alone.

I would spend hours and hours thinking to myself about the universe and how it had started, and our place in eternity.

To me religious ideas were important, because I needed a standard with which to live my life, and my Catholicism provided that basis.

It still does today.

So, I believe in life everlasting, which makes it easier for me to say good-bye to a loved one.

Henry Scott Holland (1847-1918) said 'Death is nothing at all. I have only slipped away into the next room. I am I, and you are you. Whatever we were to each other, that we still are.'

He goes on to say, 'Life means all that it ever meant. It is the same as it ever was; there is unbroken continuity.

Why should I be out of mind because I am out of sight? I am waiting for you, for an interval, somewhere very near, just round the corner. All is well.'

This quotation is taken from a little card which my husband bought for my children when I was first ill, and no one knew what was wrong with me.

But it cheers me up now.

Now I am no longer confused about my graduation and my mother's death.

I triumphed to graduate when I did, and my mother was truly pleased I had got it as I said to her.

So, she could pass away into the next room, and die in peace.

I had proved myself, and that would be fine.

But I wish it had not been so.

Also, when I had my miscarriage, I wish it had not been so.

Sometimes we need to look inwards to give ourselves time and space to breathe more easily.

I mentioned earlier that it seemed like an anniversary, and so it was.

My son was graduating from his English honours course at about this time, and maybe it was the association of ideas, I don't know.

I thought maybe subconsciously that as my mother died when I graduated, maybe the same pattern would repeat itself.

It became quite strong in my mind, and I had to fight against it.

It was almost as though my job was done, to have raised my oldest child.

But this was wrong thinking.

I have two children, and my daughter has just completed the first year of her course.

And life goes on after university and after graduation; in fact it is a starting point.

We are not redundant just because our children are grown up and independent.

No, it is their starting point in life for independence, and we need to be at the ready.

Life is not easy when you are starting out, and you need all the help that you can get.

I want to be there for my children throughout their early independence, and for as long as they need me to be there.

Not like my own life where I was there on my own.

But we all do the best we can, and I hope to have this extra gift of time.

Journaling

My daughter suggested I write a journal, and I took to it to save myself.

I had been feeling pretty desperate, lots of inward thoughts, many feelings of isolation and depression, and it took me all my strength just to get up in the mornings.

So my daughter suggested I write about things I wanted to do and try and change my behaviour in that way, a bit like cognitive behaviour therapy for myself.

So, she gave me a present of a beautiful flowery diary one day and I started writing in it.

Just my thoughts, because I always found it difficult to stick to the actions, I needed to work out my thoughts.

She even sometimes left me a message in it, just to encourage me.

It did encourage me, and so everyday I got into the habit of writing a little, just a little, about whatever came into my head.

I felt that I had achieved something to be able to write, a medium which I am well used to.

At the time, I could not read more than a few words, because I could not concentrate.

But somehow with writing the words could come out a lot more easily.

Not great chunks of writing, but paragraphs.

Sometimes I would write a few sentences in the morning, just to get me going, to feel that I had

some continuity, and then look again at the words
later in the day.
But, I did not write the journal to read it back to
myself, rather I used it.
My purpose was to write down in black and white
some of the thoughts that were going round my
head.
Just to do that helped me to clarify what it was I was
thinking about, and whether I needed to do
anything about it.
Usually, it was my thoughts about the past, just
going over what I had done, and what I now felt
about earlier actions, or events which had happened
to me, especially when I was a child.
Getting the ideas out from my head, onto paper,
helped relieve the burden of them rushing round
inside my head.
It eased the anxiety I felt about having to look again
at all these matters without being able to change
anything about the past events.
It was necessary somehow just to re-evaluate what
had been done and how I perceived these things.
I must say that journaling has proved successful for
me and enabled a framework for expression and
exploration.
I have taken to journaling, not for the sake of
writing, but to order my disorganised thoughts and
progress my feelings.
Yes, I would recommend it to others.

One Wheel on My Wagon and I'm Still Rolling Along

In the words of the Lee Marvin song, life goes on
We may have lost a bit of momentum, but the wagon still rolls.
In strictly logical terms, it may seem impossible for us to roll on one wheel,
But, after all it's only a song, and we are allowed some poetic licence.
Yes, life rolls on from week to week and month to month, and year by year.
We need to remember that to assess the progress we have made.
The record goes on ….. 'those Cherokees are after me, but I'm singing a happy song'…..
Sometimes it is really hard to be able to sing, even at all.
That's where it helps to be able to listen to music and words.
But it's also important to be able to do.
This is the difference between moving on and staying still.
When you feel really tired and depressed, it is often enough just to be.
How hard that is to just be, in one place at one time, and take that in.
Anthony de Mello gives us a quote, 'your job is to be just to be'
Which is I think taken from some mystical eastern philosophy.

And which serves us well here in the western world.
Too easy it is to get carried away with the latest
whim, or be drawn along in the push and pull of the
media world of excitement.
Then, it is necessary just to be, in the peace and
solitude of the place.
When you have enough confidence in being, then
you can understand what it is like to be a human,
being.
Being human is a state to understand, and we are all
human in our distinct ways and styles in this diverse
culture.
Peace be with you, is a very comforting phrase.
When we have learned how to be then we can move
on to do.
And of course human beings need to do.
In the modern economy, it is usually a question of
having a job, so it is necessary to get up in the
morning and get out to work.
This in itself is hard enough, so it is often easier to
start off by doing some voluntary work, where the
motivation comes from within to be there.
Once established in voluntary work, then motivation
feeds upon itself, and helps us to reinforce that
necessary daily motivation to get up and do.
The next step from wanting to do something is to do
it.
We need and want to work so we do.
Once in work of course the motivation is there, to be
paid a wage, to take home at the end of the week or
the month for a job well done.

Perhaps there will be the chance of a promotion, or a credit for the work completed, which again fuels our desire to get in there.

So, from the position of being out of work, in despair, not knowing how to be, we can move over to that of doing a respectable job.

No matter the state of the wagon wheels, we can keep moving along.

And anyway, we have all heard of repairs being done, so we can patch up that wagon wheel, and really start rolling.

The pressures of time and the stress of modern life may be chasing us,

But on we go, knowing that we are safe by being at peace.

We learn that life goes on, and we learn to do other things to fill in for those we lost along the way.

'Yes, one wheel on my wagon, but I'm still rolling along,

Those Cherokees are after me, but I'm singing a happy song.'

Job-Seeking

Throughout my illness I have lost my confidence for job seeking, and I need to learn to ask for a bit of help to get established again.

Part of my condition thought that I would be able to get another job, so I said I was looking for work over a year ago.

The occupational therapist made an appointment to see me, to discuss work opportunities.

That was how I saw it, but it was clear I was unable to cope with work then.

So, we discussed the next rung on the ladder, which is to get into voluntary work, and for which again I needed quite a lot of help.

An appointment was made to meet up with the local volunteer bureau, with their specialist worker, who could help people who had experience of mental health problems.

So my occupational therapist, OT, took me along to the volunteer bureau, and the three of us had coffee, and talked about me and my need to get back to work.

I became tearful, after a time; because it was obvious my optimistic and rather unrealistic attitudes about work were just not on.

It was suggested that I could do some voluntary work to get me back into a work life routine, which I accepted as the thing to do.

I kept insisting that it would only be a temporary thing, because I intended to try and find paid work.

But this is part of the whole problem, because of illness, work is so hard to find.

Then there is the confidence needed to apply for the job, and the stamina required to follow all this through.

It is a bit like steps.

One step can lead to another, but we have to be careful not to fall.

If we go too fast, we may trip.

If we go too slowly, others may overtake us, and we are left alone on the steps when everyone else is suited.

So, steps, and taking them in the right order is very important.

Voluntary work is a vital step into employment, because it gives us the time and the space to recover that necessary composure, and also a taster in the field in which we have chosen to offer our services.

I started off doing 2 days a week with the national charity Crimestoppers Trust, which has their HQ in Morden, just up the road from where I live.

They gave me a computer, and a desk and a drawer with my name on it.

All of this was very important to me, because I felt quite unsure of myself on first starting out there after my bout of depression.

You cannot really understand depression unless you have experienced it yourself.

It is so hard to describe.

It is a bit like finding yourself in a well, deep down underground, with no light and no contact with civilisation or people who might be trying to reach you to help you.

It is so important to try and stay in circulation, and doing voluntary work helps you with that.

It gets you out of the pit and helps you to maintain contact.

You are not isolated, because you are in weekly contact with people in a routine, whether it is an office, or a shop, or just some work space like a centre where people provide teas, coffees and light snacks.

You feel part of a team, where you are contributing to the general good, and your work is necessary for the end product of the whole.

You pick up on the energies and there develops a synergy, of which you are part.

Some of the workplace energy feeds into you, which helps with maintenance, or even development of your goals.

It's like the steps, one small step into voluntary work …

Then …

Who knows?

It is so important for morale to keep up with the voluntary work.

Even when there are days or weeks when you are feeling so awful that you do not want to go in.

It is vital to make that effort.

This is where it is important, not to do too much at once.

It is no good going up two steps at a time, because you may fall.

Steady, sure progress is the thing.

Building up a regular routine of the voluntary work, with perhaps some other regular social event is important.

This regularity I think is the key to getting on track, and getting back to a way of working.

After some voluntary work, you may start to feel as I did, a bit better, and more like seeking paid work.

So, you may think of the various schemes that there are to get paid work.

There is the benefit trail to follow too, and you can be on incapacity benefit and still earn some money, by being in part-time work, so it is worth while finding out about.

I phoned up and made an appointment to see the specialist disability officer at the department of employment.

She saw me and explained about the various schemes there are.

In particular there are two ways you can get help with finding work.

One is that you can go to specialist centres where they help you with skills training and preparing CV's until you can get a job.

The other is where together the specialist worker and yourself meet and talk about the job opportunities and she can help smooth the way.

It may be possible to arrange a specialist time of going in to the office, on a part-time basis initially, to try it out and to see if you can get on.

This can help ease the way in a number of different ways.

It can increase your confidence by going in on a part time basis, to see how you get on.

There is not the pressure, as if you were going in to the job full time.

This gives the employer and yourself time to adjust and see yourself in the role ….

I can see so many benefits to this.

Because you can still keep up your voluntary work at the same time, on the other regular days.

This ensures that you keep that stability there as a necessary pre-requisite for your return should the job not work out.

There are also schemes sometimes run by local MIND groups, in conjunction with health authorities, who want to see people getting back in to work, and in support of those with mental health difficulties.

It is my belief that these mental health problems can be lived through and worked through, and eventually we can come out the other end.

Job-seeking is an important area to consider in this process of rehabilitation for mental health service users.

Chapter 23 - Psychiatrist's Report

I asked my psychiatrist for a report detailing his involvement with me as a patient, explaining that I intend, as I had suggested to him when I sent him the Poems For Mental Health, to publish my account of my experiences, because I think it is therapeutic for me, but also because I know from other available books that it is useful for people to read other relevant accounts of their illnesses. Too many are sensationalist and overstated. Let us concentrate here on reality. To start with I gave the psychiatrist a copy of the first draft of my book, and asked the deputising psychiatrist to hand him the copy for him to read. He did promise that he would discuss my needs for the book with me.

My psychiatrist, Dr. Leon Rozewicz wrote, by letter of 11th December, 'I wish you luck with this enterprise.' He also sent me a Treatment Summary report dated 10th December 2003, which I reproduce here.

'Anne was first referred to the Wimbledon Community Mental Health Team on 8th January 1998. At that time, she appeared to be suffering with a depressive illness and she was commenced on treatment with Fluoxetine (antidepressant) at a dose of 20 mg a day. Because she was agitated we have also added Risperidone (this is a major tranquiliser) at a dose of 2 mg a day.

Anne's condition responded well to support and to regular sessions with our Community Psychiatric

Nurse, Don Mulvey. We were able to discharge Anne completely from our care about 6 months later.

Anne became depressed again towards the end of 2001 and we saw her again on one occasion.

Anne became unwell again in May 2002. She had become agitated and tearful. Fortunately, she again responded to treatment with Prozac and Risperidone.

Since the middle of 2002, it has become clear that as well as being depressed, there are times when Anne is elated and agitated.. We have therefore changed the diagnosis to one of Bipolar 2 Disorder. Bipolar 2 Disorder is a mild form of Bipolar Disorder with episodes of elation which do not amount to manic illness, which requires inpatient care. Subsequently, Anne has responded well to treatment with Risperidone and the antidepressant Venlafaxine. She is currently on Risperidone 2mg a day and Venlafaxine at a dose of 150 mg a day.'

I have been gradually building up to the point where I could say to myself that I needed to take a stand again in the world. I have been hiding away in the family for the past few years with only a few forays out into that wider network. Why? Because I have been through a roller-coaster of emotions and feelings and have felt totally unable to move outwards into either the workplace or the bigger picture of the world. My world has been quite small and insular, of necessity. I have felt the need to concentrate on myself at home, to take the time to rebuild myself and my persona. It feels like I imagine trauma to be. The experiences of psychotic delusion and mania have been quite mind expanding, although horrific and terrific at the same time. I always knew I was ultimately safe because I felt safe at home, but my thoughts go out to those people going through similar experiences to myself without the security of a safe home environment. However the experiences of depression have been very debilitating. The hours spent crying, the days spent without the motivation to even get out of bed until late, the lack of purpose to any part of the day, without direction from another. Oh the feeling of utter desperation, with no feeling of ever getting out of that hole. I do not say this lightly at all either, and it is no good people saying she just needs to pull herself together, because it was just not possible. I am one of the lucky ones, one of the survivors in these episodes of manic depression. You only need to read some of the other autobiographical accounts to realise that so often despair sets in and a chasm envelops the sufferer. Many are the times I have sensed this feeling, but I have always had my husband to pull me back up and out of this terror. I wrote an article once called 'Help with Pulling Yourself out Of Depression'. I reproduce it here now in case it is of help to anyone. I wrote it when I was feeling very low, and I felt there was little of cheer in my life, apart from my family, except for the church group which I attended once a week on a Thursday. The parish priest had invited me along to the prayer group originally set up for people with mental health difficulties, and at the time I was in a desperate state. Again, I have regularly attended this prayer group once a week over the last year, and I feel it has helped me greatly. There never was any pressure to attend at all, it was totally voluntary, but for some time it was the only thing which I could attend, and I could carry on going there whether I felt well or not. The mood of the group and of the organisers was always supportive and non-judgmental, so that was a great welcome. It was after attending one of their meetings that I wrote this article. Here it is:-

'It has been likened to being in a deep dark well where you see nothing, except if you are lucky, maybe a glimmer of light above. There is no one else there. You are all alone. It is blackness all around you, with no landmarks, or signs or helping hands. It is like being blind, because you can see no-one. Yet there you are. But where is it? Where are you? When you get to thinking about it, it is very scary, because maybe for the first time in your life there seems to be no structure. There is surrounding emptiness, and an eerie silence, except for perhaps the wealth of thought pounding

*round your own head. Why is there no-one there,
beside you? Where is everyone else? Who are you?
How do you know who you are if nobody is talking to
you or with you, or seems to understand you and how
you are feeling?*

*Again, imagine that at the top of the well, on the
outside there are people there, although you cannot see
them. These individuals and groups of people will be
looking down, but cannot see you, not because they
cannot see, but because it is so dark, and such a long
way down. That does not stop those helpers at the top.
No they remain there; they are there, straining to see,
to detect any movement, or positive signs of energy
below. It is like a chasm, and an open void below them,
and they often have no real idea of how to make contact
with the individuals trapped below. But they remain
there in hope and love. This group includes
professionals, carers, family members, friends, social
groups, charities and other concerned members of
society, like clergy and parish members. What tools or
mechanisms do they use to find out who is struggling
below? Therapies, counselling, medication,, treatment,
social visits, befriending services, support groups,
spiritual help, church involvement, encouragement, and
direct help like listening, going for a walk together,
exercise, sharing a meal, spending some time together.*

*Where are you though, for sometimes I cannot see you,
I am so locked into the darkness below? I feel tired and
think I need a rest, but the thoughts keep me anxious
and worried about all sorts of troubles which face
many of us at different times in our lives. "Out of the*

depths I cry unto you oh Lord, hear my voice. Let thine ears be attentive to the voice of my supplication." Prayer is an important communication tool, and is always available to us, either individually, or in small groups, or at the larger church services. Meditation and prayer groups are there for us, to share our time and different ideas about the gospels, and stories or passages for meditation. Have you thought of going to one? Have you thought of making that time for God and also for yourself?

It is hard to find peace, but we are all searching for our different paths. "Be still and know that I am God." The other day I was singing when I came home, and the tune 'Be still and know that I am God" kept running through my head. I felt joy, which replaced the often melancholy thoughts and anxieties which seem to keep me occupied each day. So how did this happen? What had I been doing? Would I recommend it to others? I had attended a small prayer group meeting with my local parish priest, invited along after talking about my feelings of depression. Mental health is a gift – make sure you treasure it – far too often our lives get out of balance and priorities are distorted. Yes, I try to be positive, and to make a note of my achievements and to value those of my family too. But life can be hard when you have depression, both for you and your family, your carers and friends. So, it is important to be positive and try and find a way forward, depending on your circumstances. It is crucial to have a balance in your life, with spirituality featuring in the list of factors, along with health, exercise, self, work, family and friends, etc. How often do we take time out and make time for spiritual prayer, meditation, spiritual readings. To me, this is all in addition to the various examples of voluntary work which many of us get involved in the parish and beyond. What was special for me about this spiritual group which I was invited along to, was the regular attendees all welcomed the newcomer, and I was introduced to the regulars. We spent half the time in a collective prayer and gospel reading and were invited to pray and meditate on the passage. Various issues came up quite easily, and there was time to pray for our own intentions. A feeling of peace came to the meeting – there was no pressure, and our stresses of the day had been left behind. The joyful mysteries were mentioned, and after the concluding prayer we all shared a cup of tea or coffee and a slice of cake. It was a real tea party, like I remember from oh so many years ago. There was plenty of social chit chat helping us to enjoy the occasion. At the end of the hour our time was up, and we made our way home. I felt inspired to go swimming, then headed home singing in my head 'Be still and know that I am God', and then to write this short article for others to read."

My daughter once suggested to me that I take up journaling, and the idea of it appealed to me immediately. She gave me a lovely little notebook with pretty, colourful pictures of flowers on the front, and a neat compact size which I could easily hold in my hand. She helped me with it by writing a response to the first pages of writing which I put in, and gave me lots of kisses. This little notebook is a precious possession, and I really valued its existence to keep me going. When I was ready to do something in the day, I got my little notebook, and started writing about how I felt. It got me going, because sometimes it is just impossible to think of doing anything at all when you have depression. But, to go to my notebook and write gave me satisfaction, especially knowing that it was a present from, and an idea from, my daughter. No one else had come up with suggestions of what I could or should do, that I felt I could manage. When my notebook was finished, I bought a large exercise book with A4 size pages, and wide spaced lines, so that I had a framework for writing. I used this over the next year, and its two successors, to get a stand on my life. I sometimes found it helpful to copy out large chunks from books I was reading, which I felt were particularly pertinent to my life. Also, if I was unable to read or concentrate, as quite often was the case, I could just take my pen and write about how I felt unable to concentrate or think and I would ask God for help. Just putting pen to paper helped me, because although I was unable to do anything else, when I had written a few lines or a few pages, then that meant I had achieved something. Also, later in the day I could see the progress I had made by referring to the feelings I had had, and how I felt then. Sometimes I would take to writing again in my journal, particularly if I was feeling anxious. I must say that I have endured many, many years of feeling anxious, and it has been an incredible strain for me, always worrying and feeling nervous about what was going to happen.

When I think of all the experiences I have had because of my manic depression then I realise it has shaped me in my ability to deal with other people's feelings and experiences of depression and mental illness. Prior to my own suffering I would feel scared of mental illness as a condition and felt I had nothing to offer those people who were stuck in depression. Now I feel I can be far more positive about it, and if I identify someone else who has experienced depression there is an instant rapport, often leading to friendship. Many times I have thought it would be a good idea to set up a system of self-help support in this area of need, and all it needs is the opportunity.

Chapter 25 - Writing This Book

Perhaps this book is one of the really positive steps which I have taken off my own bat. I think it has really grown out of my use of journaling, and is as I see it a natural extension. I think I will introduce you here to some of my journaling writings over the last year. I will list them chronologically, so that the reader can see that there is really no natural progression to my writings. Rather, this shows the nature of mental illness, the ups and downs which can be quite difficult to deal with. This is not a complete reproduction of my journaling by any means – I filled a lot of exercise book in a period of less than a year, when the need to express myself in writing was strongest. Sometimes a week would pass when there were no entries, and other times there may be two or three on the same day. It would reflect my need to express myself, and of course you, the reader, must remember that I would be largely alone in the house during the day, so without conversation, writing seemed a natural way to make my feelings known. And it was important for me to express my feelings, because otherwise the thoughts would just go round and round my head.

I started off my journal on 22nd October 2002 with - I have been medically diagnosed as having depression. I am on prescribed medication of Prozac and I am desperately trying to get back my positive attitude to life. I was first put on Prozac about six years ago when I went out of my mind with worry. I had been working round the clock for many months, helping my husband wind up his business, my son who was 16 years old at the time thought he had a brain tumour and was dying, and my step-mother had recently died, after a relatively short illness. I was so tired emotionally, I could not hold on to where I was. I even prayed that I should have my son's brain tumour, so that he could be saved. In the meantime, our family life, with two adolescent children, and no paid employment immediately in the offing for my husband, continued, until I could no longer cope. I became ill and after a bit of a time on a tranquiliser, Valium, after seeing the psychiatrist I started my term on Prozac with Risperdal.

Now six years later, I am still on Prozac. I have been off it twice, trying to manage my life without this drug. Most recently again, I was on a dose of Risperdal morning and evening, which lasted for 4 months, and had me feeling like a zombie, physically exhausted and mentally cut off. I was desperate to get off this drug, especially when I started feeling I was useless, and even my mind entertained thoughts of it being better for me to be dead. I had never felt that way before. I was very scared to be on a drug which had been prescribed for me, yet to feel so isolated, detached and alone. I saw the community psychiatric nurse at this time, but that did not alleviate my concerns. When I look back now at that time in July and August, some two months ago, I can appreciate I have made a great deal of progress, for which I am especially grateful. In my particular case I knew I had to hang on to who I was, what I had done, and to my achievements, which included raising two children, now aged 19 and 22, a daughter and a son, with my husband.

Later in the day I wrote: I've been spending time reading meditations from Anthony de Mello's 'Taking Flight' and 'Song of the Bird'. There are lots of useful references and ideas and here is an important one about learning 'to be'. "Your duty is to be. Not to be somebody, not to be nobody – for therein lies greed and ambition – not to be this or that – and thus become conditioned – but just to be." It's easier to read a few sentences and then think about them for a while when your concentration is poor, and your mind is racing, unable to focus on the words on the page, or read any other kind of book. So when my head was busy I had to spend a lot of time just thinking, because my body felt exhausted and would not move much. At the time I was zonked out on Risperdal I would watch the clock and watch time pass from one hour to the next, sometimes from one five minute stretch to another. I was lucky to be able to find the energy to walk 5 minutes along to the supermarket to buy the food for the evening meal, and a little household shopping. Everything was minimal. There were no new recipes or interesting casseroles to eat. The family were lucky if I put some potatoes in a pot, or opened a pack of cold ham and made a simple salad. Often my husband prepared a meal, or my son or daughter. I felt very guilty, and that I ought to have done the meal properly, but I was totally unable to do any more. Last year I wrote a paper called 'Improving Mental Health in the General Population' and I even sent it to a Community care magazine for publication, but was told they could not take it. That did not stop me, because I prepared two other chapters and sent it through to a women's press unsolicited. In these days of stakeholder involvement you would have thought that my written contribution would be welcome and useful at some of these professional magazines, or meetings held by community groups.

Later in the day I wrote: Today I went by appointment to the Volunteer Bureau, with the Occupational Therapist. I would not have gone without her accompanying me – I put on a brave face. We met the specialist volunteer co-ordinator who works specifically with people with mental health difficulties. The idea is to give specialist support to volunteers who have depression and other mental health problems like me. It was quite comforting to be offered help like this – she will actually come to the suggested workplace and introduce me and explain a little of my difficulties, so that I have a proper point of contact and true understanding of my condition, and my need for support. Yes, I need to go with this; I need help and support like all the people I have helped in the past. That's OK. I feel vulnerable and sometimes seem to have a disability – it is so variable. The Occupational Therapist dropped me back at home and then said that was the end of her involvement, so she would notify my GP and that would be it. OK. So alone again. I did say at the interview to both the workers that there was nobody to talk to. I have already contacted the Pastoral Care Foundation asking for someone to befriend me. I read their leaflet that they befriend – listen, chat, talk and sometimes accompany to an outing. I would really like somebody to talk to, someone I can tell about my feelings of loneliness and isolation at this time, and they will be there for me and befriend me. I was also told about their volunteer support group and I asked to be invited along to that. Perhaps meeting others in the same situation as me would help.

In the last couple of weeks I have been making a determined effort to throw out my hands for help and to do things that have presented and seemed right. David has taken me swimming and about four weeks ago we started back at yoga. This is really good for both of us. Before this I just felt so desperate. Coming off Risperdal was like hell. I would be in tears and floods of tears, I could not settle, I would roam around the house or else take to my bed, feeling awful. David would phone me 3 times a day. I told one good friend and she came round to see me, then the following week I went round to see her. But of course she was brilliant. She has trained as a counsellor and she is my friend, so she knows how to help me by listening and by being there for me. So many people just don't know – they get fed up if you're quiet, fed up if you say anything about your feelings, and really can't cope with the threatening behaviour. By this I mean behaviour which threatens how they are and how they feel, because really they do not want to be challenged or even to have to think about how they are. My friend encouraged me to think about humanistic and behavioural type counselling, and lo and behold, about 3 days after I contacted Marriage Care they phoned to offer me and appointment for my husband and I, and we have been going weekly now for 4 weeks – 5 tomorrow.

So that was a long entry for 22nd October – they are not all so long and so involved, and I do not always write every day. On Wednesday 23rd I wrote about a phone call and a local meeting on mental health services that I had heard about. My own psychiatrist was to take part. 'Yesterday afternoon I popped into the library to see if I could find any useful books about humour, or a tape about humour. The OT told me she had heard of a group run about 5 years ago, but nothing currently. I have a real worry about my sense of humour. I used to like a laugh, but now it's so rare. Last night I did laugh at a poem that Pam Ayres was reciting on the radio about 'Just Ask My Husband' I think it was called. He was a bit of a know-all, and people avoided coming round. Oh dear God help me to move forward and to understand life. I do feel I have been in a state of arrested development, because of the trauma of my teenage years. When I think back, it is just so sad, so sad, and really I have not grieved properly at all. Before my mother died she used to feel sick, and was isolated at home, and depressed, though she tried to carry on. She had had 3 heart attacks at least, and was hospitalised lots of times. Our life was sad and lonely. Our dad was there, but I do think that a lot of the burden fell on me. My mum had a heart attack first just about a year after her own father died, and I remember how he had lived with us, and been a part of our family too. Also, our grandparents in Scotland too, they were a large part of our family life, because we went to Scotland every summer for our school holidays, and stayed with them, and then they joined us for the month of September. But there is only so much life and living you can do before life says you have had too much loss and you need to stop. Loss is a cumulative thing, just like David says convalescence is. Dear God help me to convalesce and to get better. Perhaps if I understand more about why I am like I am, and why eventually loss broke me down, then I will be able to deal with it and cope again. I found a book in the library called 'An Anthology for Those Who Grieve', called 'All in the End Is Harvest', edited by Agnes Whitaker, a Cruse publication. Many issues of types of grief and bereavement are dealt with, and on reading through the ideas and the poetry, I felt very moved and emotional, thinking about my mother and how she had died when I was 21. She died the day after I graduated from university and I know that was significant, I just do. I used to send her cards on a regular basis from Edinburgh to tell her how I was getting on. The nurses used to ask her what card she had got each day or two, because she received so many. Yet, I kept myself at a distance wrapped up in my studies, as a way of coping. I had no real friends, and did not go out much. I spent my time studying and I did all my work on time. Oh God how hard I worked, and then I graduated well, with a degree with distinction. But that was enough for me. I had had enough of all the studying, all the concentration on the work, trying to avoid the pain of my mother's illness. She had such a miserable time alone, a lot of the time, while my Dad went travelling with his work. She felt ill and sick. I think it was out of balance and not good. I always said to David I did not want him to work too long hours, because of what my dad did, and I tried each week, so that we had time together, on our own, which I say is absolutely crucial. Of all the couples I have known, so many have separated and divorced, it is horrendous. What a nightmare, all those people separated, and all their children living split lives with one parent or the other. Oh dear God life is hard for so many people. Is that not why I entered the job of social work and helping others, really? Is that not the whole main influence which coloured my life and made me into what I am. Is that why I chose somebody like David who would be there for me, and look after me, and care about me when I needed it. So why did it not work out that way for me. I remember he told me about his parents, and how his dad was a martinet, so that at the first opportunity David took off and that was in his early teens, when he'd go off for the weekend, and then travel the world, and also be on the go all the time. He did not really want to be at home at that time either. But since then, all through the children's childhood we have kept in close touch with his parents. David's mum always told me that he was the one son whom she never lost touch with – she would always talk to him, and she took him to the edge of Birmingham when he went off on his travels. Before David and I married I said to David's mother that he seemed such an independent person, and he didn't really seem to need a wife. David's mother said yes, he did. So I listened to her, as I always have done. David speaks to his parents, particularly his mother, quite a lot, and they do seem to have a close bond. It makes me feel jealous sometimes, because I do not have that close bond with my mother. After my mother died, I have just tried to get on with my life. Perhaps what I need to do is try and remember all the nice things that I did with my mum, and what she did for us, so that I can 'internalise' these feelings and be happy that I had a mum. Lots of people of my age now have to come to terms with the fact that their parents are ageing and dying, and they are facing bereavement, after a lifetime together. Perhaps my lifetime took place before my mum died, by the time I was 21 I was an adult and I had experienced a whole range of emotions.

When I was ill in the summer on Risperdal, I remember the whole range of emotions I went through. I wrote to David's mum saying I could not believe the wide extent and depth of emotions that we can have – it is just incredible, and also very scary indeed. Feelings are such powerful things, they can take us over, and lead us this way and that, all over the place, but it means that you feel like you are on a roller-coaster, and that cannot be good. At the funfair when I was about in my 20's I did not like the rides any more – they made me feel sick, jolting me this way and that, it was horrible. So, I learned to avoid them, and I think it was David who went on the funfair rides with the children. I do not like being jolted around, it makes me feel ill – I need to keep my life in balance so that I can think clearly, slowly and deliberately, without being pressurised into doing this or that. I need to be able to stand up on my own two feet and say that I am a good and lovable person. I have lost so much of my self-esteem and self-confidence over the last few years with illness, and I have worked overtime to support my two children. I always felt as though I had to protect my 2 children, so strongly, that it took up all my energies in the end. Of course I did not know that this was happening at the time, because I felt as though I had done something wrong, and was being punished for it, not that I was just like everyone else, and finding life itself difficult. I am just like everyone else – nothing more, nothing less. I am just an ordinary human being, doing the best I can to live my life. The hardest job of my life, raising my two children, is now finished, to a large extent, because as my children are young adults, they want to take off and go out and about and find their lives. No doubt they are anxious about their parents too, because they want them to be well, and to be able to enjoy life again. Dear God, please help me to grow stronger and more independent again, so that I may be able to offer the world, and my own family, something. I have been so dependent on David for the last few years, so 'needy', so desperate to be loved, that it has been difficult for us all. Oh I need to be loved, as I am, not as I was. I am now 51 years old, I have done a lot of things, and I have my own ideas and opinions, and I want the chance to express them, not just to be talked at all the time. Some people talk too much, and others are therefore forced into the listening, or shall I say more passive role. This is not a healthy balance. We all need to be able to speak, to talk, to listen, to have a conversation, to exchange and share views. Talk is a commercial tool, enabling us to share ideas, to move forward, not just to get information. It is about concepts, not things, and what may hold to be true at one point today, may change tomorrow, if there is fresh information, new ideas, or a new person joining the conversation. Each person has something to contribute. Each single person in life. That is why sometimes it is just your role to introduce someone to the conversation, to say this is someone who would like to say something, or has something to say, so can you make a bit of space for them to talk. Just a little, a little space. It does not

have to be more than just a few words, because maybe
that is all they need to say today.

Reading about grief and love is quite moving. "Love
than death itself more strongly." Here are a few lines
by Sir Walter Raleigh:
"True love is a durable fire
In the mind ever burning.
Never sick, never old, never dead,
From itself never turning."
Perhaps the ideal is in the end for the dead person to
become a part of you. Some of their opinions, skills,
insights, and values become inter-mingled with our
own, and in this way, leave their strongest legacy.
"Moderation in all things" is what my mother used to
say.

"A sense of continuity can only be restored by
detaching the familiar meanings of life from the
relationship in which they were embodied, and re-
establishing them independently of it. This is what
happens in the working through of grief." 'So long as
the change will be gradual enough to sustain a
continuity of meaning. Grief can be mastered, not be
ceasing to care for the dead, but by abstracting what
was fundamentally important in the relationship and
rehabilitating it. The change may be unstable, too
tragic to sustain any future. We need to formulate a
sense of ourselves, which neither rejects nor
mummifies the past, but continues the same
fundamental purposes. Until then, there may be
overwhelming feelings of disintegration." All this is
said by Peter Marris in from 'Loss and Change'. After

loss we can change, I am sure of it, so it is all a gradual process of change. Dear God help us to move ahead and change. From 'Death and the Family' by Lily Pincus. "This process of internalizing the dead, taking the deceased into oneself and containing him (her) so that she becomes part of one's inner self, is the most important task in mourning. It does not happen immediately, for a varying span of time the bereaved is still in touch with the external process of the lost person. Once the task of internalising has been achieved, the dependence on the external presence diminishes and the bereaved becomes able to draw on memories, happy or unhappy, and to share these with others, making it possible to talk, think or feel about the dead."

'Fear, face the fear and learn strategies to cope with the fearful feelings. Learn relaxation and imagination techniques at the same time, to reduce anxiety. I have always felt fear and been anxious. I have always been troubled by what could happen. Why? Who do I have to always feel anxious – I need to learn to relax, to do meditation, to take up hobbies, interesting things to do, to visualise. In the class on self-esteem we learned about visualisation. We listened to a tape on visualisation and feeling the negative feelings going out, down through our body, through our feet. That felt quite good.

CRT _ Cognitive Remediation Therapy helps improves concentration and memory, particularly for people with schizophrenia. Follow conversations, watch TV and undertake tasks. It is a form of psychotherapy and can be measured in terms of brain scan. This information was on a radio programme by Dr Raj Persaud, who is a psychiatrist and on TV too. Frontal lobe of brain is involved in this change and we can be optimistic that this will change on, with talk, rather than just meditation. Talk rather than tablets is a programme coming up on the 'All in the Mind' www.bbc.co.uk/radio 4 is the website, and could have useful information for us to check out this behavioural idea. We need to change our behaviour in order to make changes in our life. Tagore talks about 'endless harmony of pain and peace united'. Love can die in many ways, most of them far more terrible than physical death. There is opportunity for rebirth and life after death. Faith and belief help us onwards, to appreciate with 'with God be the rest'. We cannot know what we cannot know, so we trust in God and have faith. We should not speak of our love in the past tense. Love is a thing which does not fade in a faithful heart. It does not go into the past unless we betray our love. We must keep our love alive in a new situation. Our love cannot be dead because a person has died. Our life must be a continuation of theirs.'

Here is a poem 'Remember' by Christina Rosetti

'Remember me when I am gone away,
Gone far away into the silent land;
When you can no more hold me by the hand,
Nor I half turn to go yet turning stay.
Remember me when no more day by day
You tell me of our future that you planned:
Only remember me; you understand

It will be too late to counsel then or pray
Yet if you should forget me for a while
And afterwards remember, do not grieve:
For if the darkness and corruption leave
A vestige of the thoughts that once I had,
Better by far you should forget and smile
Than that you should remember and be sad.'

More information from the Cruse handbook says 'The course of mourning cannot be predicted. Patterns will vary for each individual. The process has varied norms, and there is no norm for adaptation. Life is seasons. Episodes of despair and depression may follow illness or other internal or external situations. The mourning process involves the healing of a wound. Only when the lost person has been internalized and becomes part of the bereaved, a part which can be integrated with her own personality and enriches it, is the mourning process complete, and then the adjustment to a new life has to be made. It is the part of courage, when misfortune comes, to bear without repining the ruin of our hopes, to turn away our thoughts from vain regrets. Inspiration comes from imagination. The gate of the cavern is despair, and its floor is paved with the gravestones of abandoned hopes. There self must die, so the soul can be freed from the empire of fate. The Gate of Renunciation leads again to the day light of wisdom, by whose radiance a new insight, a new joy, a new tenderness shine forth to gladden the pilgrim's heart, says Bertrand Russell. 'In time I will be tempered like fine steel to bend, but not to break', says Marjorie Pizer. A bit like non-destructive testing. Blessed are they that mourn, for they shall be made strong.

Thursday 24th October
'Rebirth' by Marjorie Pizer
'I am emerging from an ocean of grief,
From the sorrow of many deaths,
From the inevitability of tragedy,
From the losing of love,
From the terrible triumph of destruction.
I am seeing the living that is to be lived,
The laughter that is to be laughed,
The joy that is to be enjoyed,
The loving that is to be accomplished.
I am learning at last
The tremendous joy of life.'

'Acceptance' by Brenda Lismer
'There is an end to grief
Suddenly there are no more tears to cry
No hurt nor break now
But mute acceptance of what will be
Knowing that each move for good or ill
Must fit the whole
Past comprehension
Yet trusted in the design
This way lies peace.'

Friday 25th October
People live on in what they do, in their actions, in the memories of those they have influenced. Perhaps this is the key to remember the loss of my mother, and my baby who died too. We always talked about the little

baby who would have been the little life that would have been lived. My mother died 30 years ago, and the little baby 15 years ago. How time melts into one. When I look back now there is a blend of my past – it is there, making me what I am today. I have to accept all these things that have happened to me, all the grief, all the pain, all the trauma, all the hurt, all the sadness, all the feeling and emotion, whether buried or no, and trust that 'this way lies peace'. Dear God help me to incorporate all these losses and emotions into me. There have been a lot of things I have not understood, as time went on, but I did try to understand things in the way that I knew, I mean what else could I do. I thought I had to be the quiet, gentle, demure female, who always smiled, and people would like me, but that model soon became really outdated. The only problem with it was that I had nothing to replace it at all. I became sad, angry and lost. Loss leads to feelings of loss very often, unless you can find a way forward. Grief helps. I have had to postpone the grief of losing my mother, for me, because at the time I had grieved as I thought, her death before she died. To me, the sadness was there, that she was ill for years with heart attacks, in bed, then feeling sick. She did not seem to have much to do for herself, with friends I mean, she did not have friends to chat to, and a life at least outside of the home. That's why we seemed to have this past, ghastly as it is, of me working and holding it all together, me working like a bloody idiot, studying all the time, not developing friendships, just working so that I could pass my exams. Later, I always worked hard in the jobs that I did too. I heard a friend's voice yesterday saying that I probably got too involved over the years and I think that's what it is, thinking all the time that if I just gave another bit of myself, lost another bit of myself, in the general purpose of holding it all together, then it would be OK. But what I have to remember and to learn that I am only a human being. God gives me the strength to carry on, day after day, to do what he has put there in front of me. He gives us unfailing strength to bear it. And he has. When I was first ill, I felt OK. I was on medication and diagnosed as depressed but it did not worry me, I felt as though I was being looked after by David, so it was alright. For perhaps the first time I could take a back seat. The only difficulty with this is that it has been hard for him. He has learned other ways of coping, like relying on his family and now regularly speaks to his mother, particularly, sometimes his father too. This has had added benefits because he has got so close to his parents, which after all these years has been good for him. He established bonds at an early age with his brothers with whom he went travelling, and he's still running away now, maybe he wants a different companion. This is why there is a lot of pressure to go off on these 'adventure holidays'. But it is such hard work. We did all this with the children, because it was good fun for them – we did as much as we could for them, taking them on all sorts of activity holidays. The best thing to do is to remember all the best things that have happened, all the good things, and to try and respect these good things but not the bad. If we emphasise the positive, then this builds on itself. +++ This builds up and up, into a strong force. Dear God, help me to see that I have done my best within the limitations of a human body, within the limitations of my understanding, at the time, because of my particular experiences and what has happened to me in life. We are all limited human beings – limited by our experiences that are all. I always thought I was lucky, and to some extent looking back now I think I was. However, love, real love, is not easy, passive stuff, love is real, love can be tough, love can say, get on with it. I'm afraid that I had too much of the entire passive stuff – far too much. Love is patient and love is kind, but love is not passive. That's why you could even say that a couple who have an argument are showing they care – they care enough to try and state their case. God, it's much worse in a horrid kind of way to be passive, not to say anything, or to pretend that life is OK, or that there seems to be no feeling. In that way there is a death, because love needs to be reinforced, love needs to grow and to be reinforced.

Watching a science and medical programme the other night there was talk about the fight and flight syndrome, and fear and taking risks. Fear is what happens when there is paralysis in the amyglada – which is where serotonin works. So, it could be said, could it not, that really anti-depressants which give relief for depression are helping to counter the feelings of fear. Maybe fear is that where the brain is running away. Fight or flight, or what is it that drives us on? Fight = anger. Flight = fear and in the longer term can lead to the chronic state of depression. So, what else is it that comes into the equation of wanting to carry on? Is it self-preservation? Is it the desire for God's love, the overwhelming desire to love the Lord they God with thy whole soul, whole heart and whole mind.

Here we also learn that we need to learn to love our neighbour as ourselves. This can be hard, because we may find it hard at a particular time to feel that we are worth loving. Why is it that we are worth loving -- because we are loved by God – God created us – God made us. So, we are God's creation, and that is of the highest order. God made us to know him, love him and serve him in this world and to be happy with him for ever in the next. So, spirituality and our spiritual life are there for us, and needs to be developed. It is not enough to call to God in our misery, rather we need to trust in God and live a spiritual life. This takes time, to pray, to learn to talk to God, 'to be', to be in God's presence too. A prayer groups helps with this – we learn 'to be' with others, we learn to share our time, and ourselves. We learn that we all are on a journey of love. It is quite a long and tiring journey isn't it, but not as hard as that of Jesus Christ, who was beaten, humiliated, stripped of his clothing, and found guilty at a trial, then made in the weakened state he was in, to walk carrying the cross to which he would be nailed and would die. Our Good Friday, our Resurrection, these will happen too. Many people have been put to death throughout the world, starved through lack of having proper agricultural policy, and the unfair distribution of human resources. We need to change the world, and we need to change ourselves. By keeping ourselves on the path, getting back on when we have fallen off, trying again, helping others along the way, like Simon of Cyrene, who helped Jesus directly and openly. The path is difficult – we may fall off and need to get back on. We are talking about the path of perfection, trying to find the way to God. We are not perfect though, we make mistakes, we take the wrong path, we get lost, and we find ourselves in the wrong place, sometimes without even knowing anything about the journey. Here we are one day – we wake up here. But where is it? Where are we? And who are we? We may feel we are at the bottom of a deep, dark well, and we may feel that there is a veil over us. How can we lift it – is it heavy, or is it like a web, that seems to stick like glue. Does it just bind us up further and further, so we become fully covered and tied up by this veil? Maybe we can't even see through it at all. Perhaps we are trapped behind it. God knows it all. Not even a little sparrow falls without God knowing. The same with being at the bottom of a deep, dark well lost inside. There may be people trying to help us on the outside but we can't see them when we are below. We are lost in the dark, like lost sheep. Why are we there? How did we get there? It is just such a tragedy to be lost there. God help us all. Please help these people who are above, looking down to help us, to see us in the dark, to offer the right kind of help.'

Saturday 26th October
Returning to fear, there are two named parts of the body where fear takes hold – according to the programme. One is the brain and the amygdala, and the other is the liver, where again so far as I understood it, it is again paralysis. Action or inaction. "To be or not to be." To do shows what action we can do, and have done. It is important to do. By doing, it helps us to be. We cannot possibly spend all our time reading or talking. It is much better to do something. This may be slow, and step by step, but at least it is doing. Far

better that than giving up and not doing anything. So, for example, spending time exchanging conversation is good, making clear our needs is important, and making instructions clear. Doing journaling is again, a useful skill, because it helps us to 1) spend time doing something positive – we can see the physical result in written pages, 2) helps externalise our feelings by writing down what otherwise would be purely internalised thoughts, unless we spend time sharing our ideas with someone else, or a group, 3) reduces isolation. By help with focus, and concentration we can help ourselves tune in to what others are thinking, e.g. by listening to the radio, and taking notes, or by copying out a poem, or by writing our thoughts in a constructive way, 4) it helps impose a sort of a discipline to our day too. We could journal at a set time, or we could make the time to sit down quietly, after a busier time, we could sit and write, 5) by writing, by doing, it is a task, which maybe stops anxiety and our thoughts wandering abstractly, or in an indeterminate way, merely because we have to command our thoughts to pen the sentences together.

Relaxation and meditation are also important for a balance of mind and body. After a lifetime so far of rushing around being busy, physically, I have been trying to change the whole balance of my being. Breathing in a regular manner, in/out, in/out, rhythmically, over time, initially for a minute or two, and increasing to a longer time of ten or twenty minutes helps us again focus our attention over a period of time. Combine the relaxation technique of breathing with movement, into a sort of rhythm of exercise is what yoga seems to be about. It is an alignment of body and mind together. We learn to move and to inhale/exhale at set times in the physical process of movement and breathing and so to control our output. We learn balance; we can see whether we can physically stand on one leg, looking at a set point, and whether we can do this on both sides of our body, both left and right. It is amazing how different everyone is. In yoga classes, we do a range of movements and exercises, and because everyone's body is different, we have a different range of ability. I like yoga because it is non-competitive – we work with our own body – we go at our own pace – we gradually improve as we strengthen in mind and body. In order to prepare for a yoga class it is best to be casually and coolly dressed, and free to move. At the end of the session, when there is final relaxation, it is important to keep our body warm for the ten minute slot, so either wear more clothes or take a blanket. We need to be warm in body to be able to relax – not hot, not cold, but warm. Previously, I always used to be too hot, so I took the opportunity of cooling down at relaxation. Now I seem to be less hot in body when the session is finished, but nicely warm, and exercised. I can now feel that parts of my body have been working and that there has been a stretch, which is good. The meditation class I have been attending for an hour session, is to me very similar to the yoga. I do not find the relaxation in the class that hard, so I can appreciate how it is that we can eventually get to a state of meditation. It has been described as a visualisation of inner peace, breath following breath, and thoughts following the breath, to the point where the thoughts go and the breath is there. Eventually some people have an out of body experience, and can feel as though they are sitting looking down at their body motionless. The idea in sitting still is that we get to the point where we cannot feel our body, so that by concentrating on the breath, breathing into areas of our body which feel sore, or stressed, can help reduce any physical awareness, so that our body is just there, but our thoughts go in and out of our brain. We try to control the movement of our thoughts again by the breath. If thoughts come into our brain we can acknowledge them, then they can go. If we want peace, we need to try and reach a state where our thoughts have been acknowledged and are now quietened. It is a process of peace, breathing for peace, and relaxation. It is a set time where we can escape the reality of the normal hustle and bustle of life by sitting still and relaxing, and over time with practice, get to a state of meditation. It is a means of focussing our mind, and finding quiet time again.

There was an interesting discussion on the radio, a psychoanalyst talking about our guilty pleasures, and the 4 different areas explaining why we might like to watch or not watch certain films, which give us guilty pleasures. (1) Sex, (2) violence, (3) attachment, sadness and loss, (4) childhood/childlike themes. Sometimes people like to watch films together, e.g. mother/daughter, or father/son, because it reinforces bonds, or reminds them of good times. We may enjoy films about sadness and loss, because it allows us to get in touch with our emotions, which may be usually hidden, or difficult to deal with. Sometimes we may enjoy watching sex films or people getting together through sex, because it is pleasurable. The fourth category of childlike/childhood likes reminds us of our favourite and special times, and it could be a trip down memory lane. It would be much more difficult to try and repeat exactly what the psychoanalyst said, because I was writing this paragraph after the talking had finished. Therefore it was a recollection of ideas, of concepts, and obviously coloured by what I had taken in, or not, as the case may be. It is interesting how our interpretations can vary from the original. That is OK. It is still valid. We do not have to all slavishly accept the same interpretation of facts, and someone like a psychoanalyst can accept the huge amount of variation that there is in human thought, interaction and opinions. When I was a child I thought like a child, and now I am an adult, I have to think like an adult. That means with my own identity I have to have my own opinions. When my identity has been threatened, or I've felt insecure, my opinions have been lost. I want to develop my thinking. By journaling this helps – this is a quiet way, by writing. I want to develop my opinions, by listening to the radio, by hearing what other people are saying, and by having something to say when I am invited in to a conversation. I want to be able to hold my own in life, not present as this depressive person, who one minute can talk, and the next has nothing to say. I need to be equable. I need to get a balance. I really need to internalise what my mother left for me on a tape, 'moderation in all things'. Yet, over the years I have been more and more involved in lots of different aspects, work, looking after and protecting my children, supporting David, working in the parents association, working as a volunteer, exercise or lack of it, eating or too much of the wrong thing, and drinking alcohol instead of tea or water, or finding a balance in other ways.

This leads on to the idea of too much of a good thing, too much of what initially makes me feel good, too much of what turns into a cycle of repetitive behaviour, too much of what can become addictive behaviour. I'm now convinced that there are really all sorts of addictive behaviour, which is merely a manifestation of an addictive personality's dependence on these external stimuli. It means a life out of kilter, a life out of balance, a body imperfectly balanced, addiction to short term and quick fixes, in short term gratification. But, to be truly adult we need to grow our thoughts by understanding these concepts. We need to be able to think rationally, coolly, calmly and collectedly, about ourselves and our behaviour. When we are so totally involved, up to our eyeballs and beyond, we cannot think rationally. We become emotionally charged, and there is really nothing but emotion. Equally, on the other side there is lots of exchange of ideas and information in a completely irrational, and detached way = no emotion. Again, we need a balance. We need to reduce our involvement in things like office politics, in what is going on round about us. We need to be sure of our own identity and not be shaken by all the opposing thoughts and ideas and opinions that are thrown at us. "Rough winds do shake the darling buds of May, and Summer's lease hath all too short a date", says the bard William Shakespeare.

Comedy and comedian. Comedian looks for a laugh, but the word comedy means looking to entertain. What would I rather have – it is definitely comedy. A comedian wants applause for his jokes, whereas comedy is a wider concept. Comedy, amusing anecdotes, humour, and laughter are all good, and that's what I want to learn. Firstly I need some humour and funny poems to learn, so that I know what is funny and can make me smile and laugh. Then, I need to start listening to some comedy shows, to gradually develop and to keep up with modern ideas of what makes people laugh. This could of course include topical news which keeps us up to date with the news in a straight sense, and also gives us a 'take' on how to look at it, and laugh at life. Then, I need to try and find out a bit about what humour is – what makes us laugh and how we laugh, and that it is therapeutic and why some people do/do not have a good sense of humour. I want to develop a sense of humour. I want to be able to laugh. I want to be able to join in with other people, and feel that I belong. I want and need to find out more about people and what makes them tick, and really what they are about, and how they have got to the point where they are happy, and accept their identity. When you have an identity you have a protected ego, and can go out and about and do your thing, and then return to your base having learned a little bit more. Your base gives you your sense of belonging. It's a bit like a child I think where the little child clings to the safe mother figure, and then learns to go off and explore his/her surroundings, and then can return after an adventure. Surely life really is an adventure too. We need to be able to explore life, to be awake, to be alert, and to interact with what's going on. We must not be passive. To be passive is not love, it is withdrawal. It is running away from life and real interaction. Love means caring and doing and being. Love is gentle and kind. For most marriage ceremonies we have St. Paul's gospel on love, and that is what we need to learn, to be kind, gentle, patient, and to be alive. We need to go out and meet the world, not sit back and wait for life to reach us. We have to be positive and determined. In life we need to advance, we can't be timid and rooted to the spot. We need to go forward. Soldiers in battle do not know what is going to happen, whether there are booby-traps or bombs ahead. Yet, those who have fought for us, they went forward in faith and because they believed in the cause. The cause is the rest of human race, the universe, the weaker women and children at home, who are waiting on the men who have to fight. That's why they always talked about the women keeping the home fires burning – the women making the meals, caring for the children, making clothes, keeping a routine going. Because when the men came home, they came home to an existence, a life, a country that had kept going. Because in times of trouble we need to keep going – we need to think that things will get better. We hope and pray that there will be an end to trouble and strife. No wonder so many young people got involved in campaigns like CND, Campaign for Nuclear Disarmament. After the war, life was tough for a lot of families; men came back to their wives and children as changed men. Children did not know their dads, but they had to get used to that new presence in the house, and the changed patterns of inter-reaction. No wonder many different voluntary organisations were set up to help families after the war, including groups like Marriage Care, where lay members helped the clergy deal with the problems thrown up by the long periods of separation, and the awfulness of war, fighting, death and separation from loved ones. Marriage and children are the future of the human race, so it is vital to help and support people to sustain their marriages. It is also important for those who are married to understand the importance of their role as protectors of the new young people, and to continue their work of supporting young people to grow into responsible adults, ready to take on the work of the next generation. Here is the prayer, 'We will remember them" by Lawrence Binyon.

'They shall grow not old, as we that are left grow old:
Age shall not weary them, nor the years condemn.
At the going down of the sun and in the morning
We will remember them.'

Looking up 'humour' in Brewers there is a paragraph which I now quote: 'Good humour, ill or bad humour, etc. According to the ancients there are four principal humours in the body: phlegm, blood, choler and black BILE. As any one of these predominates it determines the temper of the mind and the body; hence the expressions sanguine, choleric, phlegmatic, melancholic humours. A just balance made a 'good humour' and a preponderance of any one of the four an 'ill' or 'evil humour'.

Aggressive, assertive and people pleasing – I listened to a tape about pain and pain management. Assertiveness is in the middle. It is teaching people how we want to be treated. Body language can tell people about you. Some people do not notice body language, so you need to show assertiveness, to teach people tactfully and honestly how you really feel. It is straightforward and easily understandable. Ask for what we want – refuse to be treated without respect. We want people to modify their behaviour. Change people-pleasing and passive behaviour to assertiveness. Do not worry about people getting cross because they see a change in our behaviour. The majority of people like to see assertive behaviour. There's always a danger of rejection and hurt, but in the main people do like interacting and will thank you for a cup of tea, etc. Use the formula of 'I feel' instead of depersonalising a reaction, and coming up with words like you made me feel. Take away the idea that they have control over you. It is appropriate to be assertive when dealing with children, and we need to learn to criticise the child's action and behaviour, rather than the child him/herself. It becomes much easier to say I feel rather than stick with old behaviour. Use body language to back up your comment, and if something is funny have a laugh, or grin. Body language is important. If someone is upset or sulking, refer to this, say tell me about it so that we can sort it out, then we are giving people a chance to learn. With difficult behaviour we have a choice of putting up with it, changing it or walking away. Decide what you want to do. Allow other people to be assertive too. Assertiveness is not people pleasing; therefore consider how to be assertive, because this leads to confidence. Self esteem and happiness can follow from more direct behaviour too. So learn assertion. Pain, including stress can be relieved by relaxation. Depression can be relieved too, if looked at as a form of pain, as stress. We need to develop self-confidence and self-esteem, and get out of this cycle of pain, using it as an excuse for not being assertive.

Monday 28th October
Humour is my project. I need to try and understand more about what makes people laugh. Michael Palin who used to be in the Monty Python group is travelling through Africa and has a communication problem in the sense that the main language is unknown, therefore how does he communicate – language, noises, imitation of sounds, funny faces, repetition, slowing everything down, laughter and smiling and making others laugh and see the joke. People can understand a little this way, instead of just using words. Words/words/words – no useful communication because people can get lost in words. Actions speak louder than words don't them? Look at people's actions. Do they want others to copy or imitate them? Do they want to collect followers – do they do things for others, e.g. caressing/ cleaning/ feeding/ speaking/ doing? My mother used to like humour – she listened to the Archers, the Navy Lark, read Jean Plaidy and Agatha Christie, crime novels and Hornblower. She seemed to like books and reading. So, she would listen to the Navy Lark. So today I borrowed a tape from the Library and listened to it – it was amusing. Tony Hancock half hour was also on TV and he used to live in East Cheam (does not exist). I wish I could try and remember more about my mother – her humour – her style. Joanie seems to remember more and reads the same kind of books, and talks a lot like her. Why can't I remember more? Why is it that my experiences are so different? Oh dear God help me to remember more – not to shut it out. David is so

lucky, because he has been able to grow with his parents, both alive (until recently). For me, my life came to an early peak, and then has not been able to advance on that area, because my mother died. Her life ended – so I could no longer interact with her, certainly not as an adult and parent of my own children. I think that I have really missed out on that score. I feel really abandoned in that sense. I did try and adopt both my step-mother and my mother-in-law, because I was needy. I did not have any luck – they did not want to adopt me, because I was not their daughter. But they were companions. Oh dear God how I've felt jealous of David's relationship with his mother and his parents. I've felt locked out, and so needy, yet not able to satisfy my needs, because my model was different – it was so different. Gentle father – vibrant mother – the opposite of David's model, so he cannot understand it and runs away. Oh dear God, why did this happen?

Humour and a cup of tea en route. When we go for a walk we usually have a tea room for a cup of tea, and if it is available, a scone with cream and jam. My mum used to like a cup of tea, but she did not go for exercise. I never remember my parents going for a walk – never. I never remember outings much – occasional to the theatre, and once to the cinema or so. We spent a lot of time on our own – it was not family outings. David's family had family outings and fun holidays. We always went to Scotland, to stay with our grandparents, and only occasionally did we go e.g. to Brighton, or Bournemouth. I liked that. But again I do not remember my parents on the beach, even e.g. at St. Andrews, they stayed in the car and had soup and we had to get out on our own to walk up and down on the promenade. Oh, no, we were not much of a family for family outings in my childhood. David changed all that – he made it fun to do things for and with the children. This gave them a good childhood – lucky children, they had the opportunity to develop in childhood and they did not have the worry and emotional pressure of a mother ill in hospital. Surely they have had so many advantages and from there just have to go on and on. They enjoyed a laugh with their dad; thank goodness he has a sense of humour. Returning to this theme it seems that Newton did not have a sense of humour when he was engaged in scientific study and it was remarked that a friend did not see him laugh for 5 years when he was engaged in investigation, working hard and distracted. So, applying this theory, if we are engaged in fully encompassing work/care/study, perhaps this takes over those parts of our brain which give us relief in laughter and humour. Maybe we do not need to laugh when we are fully, mindfully occupied with life – a study or a pre-occupation. If we are pre-occupied we perhaps do not seek laughter. Perhaps laughter and humour is needed to lighten our load and help us if we are more at a loose end. Some people always seemed to be humour – fun – laughter, because they are maybe reaching out to people that way. Someone who writes a book or an article is reaching out to others and a funny book is the same. Now why did Spike Milligan, a manic depressive, on lithium, write so much? He has a number of war books, as well as books like his take on Black Beauty or Lady Chatterley or the Bible. In the Lady Chatterlay he often repeats the same joke – tying everything in together – and also his style is crude to be funny. On the Goons it is more mad lunacy of jokes/funny comments/funny voices; all interacting to amuse themselves and to make other people laugh. Take Dame Edna Everidge, who dresses as a woman (man) with glasses/hair and make up to attract attention and make people laugh. She also has jokes and stories. Jonathan Ross plays music and tells jokes and interviews people, often celebrities, so has high-powered conversations. All conversations are ways of communication – often laughs, often information exchange, often misunderstandings. Funny that – people often miscommunicate. 'What is life if full of care we have no time to stand and stare.' Time to think, time to be, time to know and time to see. If we slow things down a bit we will have time to do more. Space, lets us breathe – let's use it. I need to learn about conversation. Perhaps I should listen to chat shows, perhaps I need to listen more to the radio, and perhaps I need to practise conversations more. I do not think I'm very good at conversing now. I seem to have lost my confidence in wondering whether anyone wants to listen. Who cares about what I have to say? Hello, hello, hello – is there anybody there? Perhaps I'm just an alien landed on the planet and I don't know anything about the language.

Tuesday 29th October
I have started to read 'The Road Less Travelled' by M Scott Peck and there is a great deal of useful information in there. I have been trying to digest the text within a short time frame, so not to lose the benefit of the words; I have chosen to write some of my

thoughts down. It may not be what Dr. Scott Peck has said but rather how I take it in. The act of love – extending oneself – requires a moving out against the inertia of laziness (work) or the resistance engendered by fear (courage). In the courage of love when we extend ourselves, our self enters new and unfamiliar territory so to speak. Our self becomes a new and different self. We do things we are not accustomed to do. We change. The experience of change is frightening. Courage is not the absence of fear; it is the making of action in spite of fear, the moving out against the resistance engendered by fear into the unknown and into the future. On some level spiritual growth, and therefore love, always requires courage and involves risk. If someone is determined not to risk pain, then such a person must do without many things – all that makes life alive, meaningful and significant. Move out or grow in any dimension and pain as well as joy will be your reward. A full life will be full of pain. But the only alternative is not to live fully or not to live at all. The essence of life is change. Elect life and growth, and you elect change and the prospect of death. If you avoid the experience of death, you have to avoid growth and change. The attempt to avoid legitimate suffering lies at the root of all emotional illness. Death is our constant companion, our ally, still fearsome, but continually a source of wise counsel. With death's counsel, the constant awareness of the limit of our time to live and love, we can always be guided to make the best use of our time and live life to the fullest. If we are unwilling to fully face the fearsome presence of death on our left shoulder, we deprive ourselves of its counsel and cannot possibly live or love with clarity.

When we shy away from death, the ever-changing nature of things, we inevitably shy away from life. This is from the risk of loss. All life itself represents a risk, and the more lovingly we live our lives the more risks we take. The greatest risk we take is the risk of growing up into adulthood – a fearful leap that many people do not take. Leap into the unknown is taking destiny into our own hands. Dependency = childhood. Therapy and counselling supports and teaches courage. The extension of the self involved in loving is an enlargement of the self into new dimensions. These changes are acts of self-love. In daring to be different, even if it meant to be crazy, I am responding to earlier loving messages from my parents, hundreds of them which said, 'You are a beautiful and beloved individual. It is good to be you. We will love you no matter what you do, as long as you are you.' It is only when one has taken the leap into the unknown of total selfhood, psychological independence and unique individuality that one is free to proceed along still higher paths of spiritual growth and free to manifest love in its greatest dimensions. The highest forms of love are inevitably free choices and not acts of conformity. Commitment is the foundation of any genuinely loving relationship. There is a transition from falling in love to genuine love. Children cannot grow to psychological maturity in an atmosphere of unpredictability, haunted by the spectre of abandonment. Couples cannot resolve in any healthy way the universal issues of marriage – dependency and independency, dominance and submission, freedom and fidelity, e.g. – without the security of knowing that the act of struggling over these issues will not itself destroy the relationship. Commitment – may be beyond someone's knowledge – or neurotics may be generally aware of the nature of commitment but frequently be paralysed by the fear of it. Through death, abandonment or chronic rejection, the child's unrequited commitment to parental love, can be an experience of intolerable pain. Self-confrontation and change are necessary. But, an individual trying to grow can always retreat into the easy and familiar patterns of a more limited past. We are obliged to change and grow with our children, in order to become the parents our children need us to be. Learning from their children is the best opportunity most people have of assuring themselves a meaningful old age. There are two ways to criticise/confront another human being – arrogance, and humility. Take the second. To fail to confront when confrontation is required for the nurture of spiritual growth represents a failure to love, equally as much as does thoughtless criticism or condemnation and other forms of active deprivation of caring. No marriage can be judged totally successful unless husband and wife are each other's best critics. The same holds true for friendship. Mutual loving confrontation is a significant part of all successful and meaningful human relationships. Without it, the relationship is either unsuccessful or shallow. Leadership and power follows this confrontation. If we are to love we must extend ourselves to adjust our communication to the capacities of our beloved. Exercising power we are attempting to influence the course of the world – playing God. Love compels us to play God with full consciousness of the enormity of the fact that that is just what we are doing. There is no alternative except inaction and impotence. Self-discipline one should not be a slave to one's feelings. One's feelings are the source of one's energy. Healthy self-discipline – neither chaos nor over control. When I genuinely love I am extending myself, and when I am extending myself I am growing. The more I love, the longer I love, the larger I become. Genuine love is self-replenishing. The more I nurture the spiritual growth of others, the more my own spiritual growth is nurtured. 'Love is everywhere, I see it. You are all that you can be, go on and be it.' Love is also separateness – think of Kahil Gibrain's words on marriage.

'But let there be spaces in your togetherness,
And let the winds of the heavens dance between you.
Love one another, but make not a bond of love:
Let it rather be a moving sea between the shores of
your souls.
Fill each other's cup but drink not from one cup.
Give one another of your bread but eat not from the
same loaf
Sing and dance together and be joyous, but let each one
of you be alone,
Even as the strings of a lute are alone though they
quiver with the same music.
Give your hearts, but not into each other's keeping.
For only the hand of life can contain your hearts.
And stand together yet not too near together:
For the pillars of the temple stand apart,
And the oak tree and the cypress grow not in each
other's shadow.'

Genuine love not only respects the individuality of the other, but actively seeks to cultivate it, even at the risk of separation or loss. The ultimate goal of life remains the spiritual growth of the individual, the solitary journey to peaks that can be climbed only alone. Significant journeys cannot be accomplished without the nurture provided by a successful marriage or a successful society. As is the case with all genuine love, 'sacrifices' on behalf of the growth of the other result in equal or greater growth of the self. It is the return of the individual to the nurturing marriage or society from the peaks he or she has travelled alone which serves to elevate that marriage or that society to new heights. In this way, individual growth and societal growth are interdependent, but it is always and inevitably lonely out on the growing edge. For the most part, mental illness is caused by an absence of or defect in the love that a particular child required from its particular parents for successful maturation and spiritual growth. Healing needs the patient to receive from the therapist, at least a portion of the genuine love of which the patient was deprived. A good therapist is like a good parent. Falling in love involves a collapse of ego boundaries and a diminution of the normal sense of separation that exists between individuals. Learning and teaching – giving and receiving. Self-discipline develops from the foundation of love. The absence of love it's suggested is the major cause of mental illness and the presence of love is consequently the essential healing element in psychotherapy.

I attended session five of the self-confidence classes, tonight, so altogether we have covered emotions – feel it to heal it – empowerment, balance of life and wheel to roll. Emotions – which feelings do you habitually suppress or deny having at all. Consider how you handle each of the following emotions – openly and honestly? To yourself? Do you stuff them down? Or sit on them until you explode? Or block them from awareness? Do you handle these emotions better in some situations than others? Which feelings do you have difficulty with? Which feel more painful or scary? Which situations tend to arouse these emotions in you? What are your beliefs about these emotions?

Emotions

Anger	Compassion	Love
Grief		
Affection	Irritation	
Resentment	Happiness	
Jealousy	Hurt	
Passion	Self-Pity	
Lust	Joy	Envy
Guilt		
Sadness	Disappointment	
Enthusiasm	Shame	
	Embarrassment	
	Fear	

Where do you suppose emotions go? In what form do they re-emerge? As physical symptoms? Or feeling anxious or depressed? Or do you project your emotions onto the outside world – seeing your fears, anger, sadness or even envy in other people or in the world at large? How are your hidden emotions affecting your life? What is the price you are paying? 'To heal it, you must feel it.'

1. What makes you feel empowered? Take your power back. To whom or what do you give your power? In what situations do you hold your power? In what situations do you lose it? How do you feel in each case? 2. What do you believe other people or things can give you that you cannot give yourself? 3. Whom do you put on a pedestal? Who puts you on a pedestal? Describe the feelings and results that accompany each situation. 4. Describe truly powerful people that you know. Where does their strength lie? What do they ascribe as the source of their power? I have rights and also responsibilities. I like the right to change and grow. Someone mentioned John Cheese's book 'Life and How to Survive it'. Someone else talked about a book they had read about Jews entering a Nazi concentration camp and the author's view of the life choices he had in such a place. He said that some people in there thought they could not survive in such a camp, and within a few days quite a number of people had died. Others were determined to survive – by any means – to get out alive.

Wednesday 29th October
I have always liked the poem 'Amazing Grace' which I found today. I think they played it at my mum's funeral service, and if not, they definitely played Bach's 'Air On A G-String' – a hit in the charts at the time.

'Amazing Grace! How sweet the sound
That saved a wretch like me!

I once was lost, but now am found,
Was blind, but now I see.

'Twas grace that taught my heart to fear,
And grace my fears relieved,
How precious did that grace appear?
The hour I first believed!

Through many dangers, trials and snares,
I have already come,
'Tis grace hath brought me safe thus far,
And grace will lead me home.

And when we've been there ten thousand years,
Bright shining as the sun,
We'll have no less days to sing God's praise
Then when we first begun.'

Dr Scott Peck talks about grace, and the unconscious. There is an enormous part of our mind that is the unconscious, which we cannot possibly fully understand he says. There is the inherited wisdom of our unconscious, and it's amazing that we are actually in touch with others at all, because there is so much that is the unconscious. We need to rely on aspects of grace, of gifts from God, like serendipity and synchronicity – God gifts us these gifts in our collective unconscious, which to some extent we inherit as wisdom, and then, it is up to us to use God's gifts. E.g. we may ignore signs and messages, or we may embrace life. Dreams may throw up our unconscious experiences, as unconscious messages for reinterpretation by our brains. Love is the key forward.

Non-love is the unwillingness to extend one's self. A major form that laziness takes is fear. Risk is of the loss of the status quo. Love means risks – of extending ourselves, into new territory, new commitments and responsibilities, new relationships and levels of existence. Within each and every one of us there are 2 selves, one sick and one healthy – the life urge and the death urge if you will. Evil backfires in the big picture of human evolution. Our personal involvement in the fight against evil in the world is one of the ways we grow. An essential part of discipline is the development of an awareness of our responsibility and power of choice. The closest place to look for grace is within you. The collective unconscious is God. The personal unconscious is a place of some turmoil, the scene of some struggle between God's will and the will of the individual.

30th October

Today I went to a meditation class at 11 am then swimming and sauna on my own, and at 3.00 pm the prayer group at the presbytery. So all in all it has been a useful busy day. Humility was the theme of the Gospel, not what we show on the outside, but what we show on the inside. I told sister at the group that I was working hard to get better, and that it takes time. She made the point that if you go too fast, then you are likely to fall back, so it's day by day and step by step. I've been waiting until I felt well enough to go on holiday, as we do on Saturday, because it takes a lot of time and effort to get strong enough to cope with going away, from known bases, to explore. The word recreation – means also re-create – rebirth, start anew – as our counsellor suggested. She also asked me to leave aside the work books, counselling/personal growth and development for the holiday, and to take up some women's fiction, like e.g. Sarah Maitland and Barbara Beckwith? Browse in a bookshop and find something to suit for a light read. Today also the tickets arrived for the flight over to Nice on Saturday – the holiday is starting to happen, so that is exciting in itself. In our group, a number of people do voluntary work, and another has an interview tomorrow like me. This really does seem to be one of the major problems – occupying your time – doing either voluntary work, or paid work, and the opportunity to do so. To get up gives you a purpose to the day. Writing is a creative force – we can use our gifts to write. We can write either fact or fiction. Wouldn't it be good to write a funny book? – Now which would be an achievement for me, who finds it really difficult to tell a joke at all. But some people recently <u>have</u> said that I have a sense of humour, so I need to acquire it more and more. I need to be able to <u>grow my sense of humour</u> – it is not happiness as such – it could be a cover for real feeling, because we laugh and joke – but at least it helps with communication. And that communication can be 1:group, or 1:1 – it's often easier in a group isn't it? Because we do not have to relate at all. Whereas 1:1 we do. We need to be able to <u>share</u> our ideas. It is not for one person to do all the organisation, or one to do all the talking. It has to be <u>shared</u>. It is a bit of an exploratory thing – who is talking about what. A bit like trying to fathom what a little baby wants. A baby cries, but what does it mean?

Tired/hungry/lonely/sore? Wake up to other people
and what they are all saying there – why do they say
what they say – is it a little give-away line? Listen –
wake up to what the communication is all about. But
do not allow a take-over. Stand firm. Protect yourself.
Be like a tree in the park, e.g. Richmond Park, where
young trees are protected from the deer, which try and
eat them – barriers are put up round the tree, made out
of wood, standing round the tree, to stop the deer from
biting it. In this way the tree can grow, at least from its
early days, on to develop its self, to be going on, on its
own, at the point where it no longer needs protection,
irrespective of whether the deer are there or not. Same
perhaps with people. The parents and friends protect
young children, until the day they can stand up for
themselves. This is an important analogy.

Friday 31st October
Today I attended an 11.00 am interview at
Crimestoppers Trust – a local charity. Said I could
work on a Tuesday and a Wednesday – general
fundraising and getting sponsorship for events, etc.
They depend a lot on volunteers. They have volunteer
boards, and also volunteers in the office. They asked
me to send in a CV and also that they wanted to take up
references. God, how sick I am of having to do
voluntary work. I want a proper job, one that pays me,
so I am not dependent on people just saying thank you,
and congratulations for all the voluntary work you have
done. However, it will give me confidence. Their
office had a nice atmosphere, which I thought was
welcoming, and friendly and I said I was used to
working in voluntary organisations, where everyone

just has to muck in and help rather than say oh I only do such and such. So, my experience should be quite good, I would have thought. They seemed quite pleased too. But dear God is there not another way for me. I need to find a place where people will value me and my skills, so that I can get a proper paid job. I would have thought that with my experience I would be a good catch. Dear God, please help me to be able to get a paid job soon. Let me have a good holiday which is to start tomorrow, then to return and have opportunities open up for me. There must be a path and a way for me too. I hope so God.

Tomorrow, Saturday I set off on my travels, on holiday, so it will be unstructured – I do not know what I will find or where I will go. There are many allusions to travelling, on one's journey, like the famous books, 'Pilgrim's Progress', 'The Canterbury Tales' and more recent fairly spiritual books like 'The Journey' and 'The Road Less Travelled'. Scott Peck has also written a book about travel to find the stones, with his wife Lily. I could do a travel diary based on exploration with my husband David. Where are we setting off from? Is it Heathrow, or is it our home? We all are on a journey, but sometimes we do not appreciate we are travelling, because there are traffic jams, accidents, breakdowns, and we lose time. But time and space are in different dimensions, so, so far as I'm concerned, we can find the way again. We may lose a little time, lost like in a maze, and be unable to find our way, but eventually surely someone will find us. Luckily, if we are travelling with a partner, or with a friend, then we already have someone to help us along the way. Also, sometimes it's important that we slow down or even take a detour for another. We should not be so totally selfish – or self-centred – that we cannot listen to others. If we are on a special path together, we need to remember the decision is <u>not</u> ours alone. It is a question of communication, of talking through this point or that, through this suggestion, or that suggestion. For someone who is, or has a tendency to be, passive like me, it is important to make more of an effort. It is vital not to give up our take on life because another has, or seems to have, more ideas, more energy, or views of another. Make each day a new day, a new experience, an attempt to discover. Every day new things happen, although they are often similar to events/circumstances/ideas and conversations we may have had before. But each one is new. We need to treat each encounter as special – put time into each one, value each day, each hour, each moment, and think this is a gift. God wants us 'to be' present here now with him in the Mass, to appreciate his presence. For where one or two are gathered together in my name, then there I am too. Dear God, hear us.

Power and empowerment is important. Passion for the education of women was a very interesting programme on Radio 4 this afternoon. It was described as a rich tapestry of development – the belief of the woman behind the development was great.

I take a break from my journaling here as we went on holiday travelling around for 2 weeks in Sardinia and Corsica. I found it interesting typing this journal up now a year since it was written in pen in my exercise book. It strikes me as very intense, a real searching soul, looking to find meaning in the books she was picking up to read. What a journey through emotions, through feelings of loneliness and isolation. I remember at the time I wrote these extracts how important it was for me to do my journaling every day. It was like a hobby for me which gave me a purpose to my day. I never thought about reading the journal again a year later, and being surprised at the amount of writing I did. This is especially the case when you consider that a lot of the writing was based on readings too. But to some extent I think the journal was an occasion for me to bring up ideas which may have been going around in my head for some time. It was not all fresh new thought each day. Rather it was that my head was spinning with these kind of thoughts all the time. I had no rest from thinking. I always felt intensely about these thoughts, and to some extent it gave me some relief to be able to sit down and write about some of my ideas, out on to the paper. It was like a sort of a release in a way, writing the words down, and re-reading it all now, I can see the result of the sort of progress of my thoughts. It is a bit like as though my mind was intellectually running through lots of ideas to see if it could work things out in this process of examining my ideas. Perhaps the idea was to make progress through change, even though I was not aware of this at the time. Maybe my mind intuitively knew what it had to do, and was working without conscious prompting from myself.

I continue writing over the next year, not necessarily every day as in the October diary, but sometimes for days at a time and other times every second day. I found it a useful place also to stick in good handouts which I got from my self confidence class. I also tended to write up the good discussions which we had in group sessions, and from which I had learnt. I did a little bit of art therapy too, after picking up a leaflet in the local psychiatric out-patient clinic, which reminded me of the art work by Edward Munch called 'The Scream'. An interesting anecdote here is that once nearly 30 years ago, when I was sent to rent two art pictures to decorate the walls of an office, I chose two well known pictures which really couldn't be more different. One was this infamous scream, and the other 'Girl on a Swing' very much in Robert Louis Stevenson style. Nowadays I would still choose 'The Scream' but would find the other far too chocolate box picture-style to select. Interesting. Other interesting bits and pieces added to my journal included a couple of humorous cartoons – see I'm still working on it – and well-written, thought-provoking articles from the national papers. Such articles included one from the Care and Health magazine, on the stresses of post-traumatic stress disorder faced by war veterans, one on human trafficking and sex slavery, and how millions worldwide rallied for peace in February 2003, with the threat of war in Iraq. I also found a couple of useful leaflets again at my outpatient clinic – one on bereavement and another on understanding depression. These I read then stuck into my journal to keep them with my thoughts. I continued to write about myself and what I did, and also about changes to my medication. Here is a selection of some more journal entries, this time not a block in time, but excerpts from days here and there.

Tuesday 19th December
Took a bus to the Volunteer Bureau this morning to meet the Volunteer Coordinator at 11 for coffee. She took me into a special room at the end of the corridor. How pleasant to talk to her, she listens so well, and understands mental health issues exceedingly well. What a joy to meet up with someone else who 'understands' and is on the same emotional wave length. Further follow up meeting arranged for later in December for individual appointment, and also for 11th December for the group support meeting. Talked about my wish to eventually get paid work. Remember to start off small, as you can always increase your hours of work. Ask if I need help. Socialise, it is important to talk to others and have a laugh too. I was told about the women's drop in centre which operates on a Tuesday in the area, and how I can just go along, no referral is necessary. There is quite a lot of development going on there at the moment, and the opportunity again to do some voluntary work.

Tonight I'm going to the Self-Confidence and Development Group meeting. I'm quite looking forward to it, and feel that it will be useful for me again, after the holiday break. If I compare how I felt when the course started and now, a time span of say 7-8 weeks, then there's been considerable movement. I have indeed been making a lot of effort to develop my concentration and focus and also through the additional knowledge I've gained I do feel there's been a sizeable improvement. It is important not to go too fast – i.e. not run before can walk. It's vital to understand the need for a balance, especially where the medical profession have put it down to 'chemical imbalance'. This ties in with all my ideas of addictive behaviour – predisposition towards excess – and getting that balance right. It's like my mother said all those years ago, and it was on tape, 'moderation in all things'. That includes work. Bloody work defines so many people, which really militates against the mental health of a group in the population known as women. Women often do not have paid work and do not always work outside the home, so they are defined/ restricted/moulded and exploited by the home situation. No wonder it is women who have more mental health problems. Boundaries of acceptable behaviour are important. Remember there are outlines and guidelines which can be referred to as a protection. Excess – always running into everything can be so destructive.

I drew a picture of a triangle and marked the sides with the words child, parent and adult. Beside it I wrote where are we now? Who are we? It is a question of letting go when we have to. For example adult children need to be left alone to work out their own lives. We cannot any longer shelter, protect and encompass their egos at that stage. We need to concentrate and focus on our own needs. It is so much easier to help other people – harder to focus on our own needs. This is why we need professional support and a befriending kind of service – people to talk to, as and when we need to meet people. It is vital not to feel alone – why or why is there no-one to talk to. Talk and professional

service. I remember my local parish priest said to me –
'be' – take a minute and 'be'. He also said work out
the night before when to get up the next day. This is
important so that each day does not roll into the next.
On the other hand, if people are working then they get
up for work – that is the reason, or becomes the reason.
Many people manage because they work – there is a
structure and a routine there, which lays out the whole
approach and envelops the outer boundaries, so people
cannot get too far out of line. Whether depression is at
the bottom of a well, or on a slippery muddy slope or
trying to push uphill with a heavy weight, or e.g. a
pram, before me, then it is all isolation. Depression is
such a curse – it robs us of the day, and certainly a
fulfilled, structured day. It is so hard to get up in the
morning. Black and white rather than colour – why is it
everyone else seems to be living lives in colour and we
are on the outside in black and white. Guilt and
Catholicism may come into it, so say many people.
Change takes time. Made an interesting chicken,
onion, mushroom and potato casserole for David and
my son for dinner. They started eating as I went off to
my self-confidence class. We learned about daring to
live now, and discussed what things we had been
putting off doing that we wanted to do. Also we had to
imagine that if it was our last day on earth what is it
that we would want to do.

Friday 22nd November
I started reading the book 'The Dance of Anger' by
Harriet Learner, which was recommended to me by our
counsellor. It is a quickish book to read. It basically
talks about changing the patterns of relationships.

Think about the triangle and circular dances people do. There are so many of the different types of triangular interactions, and if they become entrenched or fixed then a lot of anger gets locked in. Remember 'I'. Remember change yourself. You cannot change people who do not want to change. So, change yourself and see the results. Others have to change, although initial resistance means that people will want you to change back. Do not. Keep with it. Also, very interestingly there are reasons why <u>particular</u> triangular relationships are set up, relating to inter-generational conflicts and unresolved issues from the first family – the family of origin, which then throw up problems for the immediate nuclear family. Birth order, death of parents, chronic illnesses and sicknesses all make their mark. Sometimes attention is focussed on a particular child – viewed as a problem – or maybe that child is merely trying to sort out the situation in the only way they know how. Culturally, women have always learned to keep their anger quiet and control it, but that's not good. Men, on the whole, like it that way. Keep ahead of time, ahead of what's going on, to be winning the battle of life. Do not run at the rear. Wake up. Jonathan Ross Chat Show in the evening had 4 guests – the actor from Jonathan Creek, David Blaine, magician and illusionist, Julio Iglesias and Miss Dynamite.

Saturday 23rd November
In the evening we attended Barb Jungar and her 3-piece woman band doing Bob Dylan songs and interpretation. His journey is long. He writes from the bus stop he is at. Grains of sand and sparrows falling. Then we went

to the Lebanese restaurant for a meal. Lovely evening. Started reading Sara Maitland's' book of short stories called 'Telling Tales'. She writes about women's experiences in historical/classical themes. There's the story of two women living alone, until the young man turns up and their whole life changes. Also the story of the twenty week miscarriage and the horror of a life that cannot be registered with the Registrar of Deaths, Births and Marriages, and cannot be buried in a cemetery. This is compared and contrasted with funeral/burial rites in four different cultures. The story of the bound feet of the Lotus blossom wife who finally could stand no more, when she saw the healthy young women and their babies in the orchard below. She remembered her childhood in the early days before age 7, when she could run around with her brothers until the women bound her feet. There is also the story of the 13 year old girl who's mother is about to give birth to the step-father's baby and compare and contrast to the freak animal museum they are visiting – also reflecting her feelings of hatred of her mother, and the mother's misunderstanding of her daughter as an adolescent. The style of writing is very erudite – many descriptive and historical words, and her strong feminist stance. She is also married to an Anglican priest.

Sunday 24th November

The article 'Memory Like Shells Bursting' is an interesting one about war and an extraordinary veteran of WWII who became a composer in his eighties. Suffering from post-traumatic stress, his condition was alleviated by the creative work of composition and music. "His imagination took flight." 'Once Norman understood that all he had to do was talk about what was inside his head or to whistle a tune, for it to be translated into music, his imagination took flight.'

Thursday 28th November
I've had a few days break from writing the journal – have been quite occupied and not felt the absolute need to sit and write about my feelings and ideas and comments. So, today I was talking to a friend who also suffers from depression, and she said she had started a journal too – one day she wrote 5 pages. Externalising our feelings gives us space inside our head to get organised. Saw a good cartoon in yesterday's Guardian paper – a large hand pointing down from the dark sky at a rather bewildered looking human being, and saying 'It's only you!' Is it God's voice speaking to us, our conscience, it's only you. Do not be afraid, just wake up to the fact it is you. Yes you. You may be small, but you can look up and realise, yes – it's me, and that's OK.

Yesterday I did the first day of my voluntary work at Crimestoppers Trust. Worked from 10-3.30, with another new volunteer, on the internet, doing searches, which I had never done before, so that was interesting. We were making new contacts for one of their forthcoming fundraising events.

Went to my last Meditation class, and got 2 handout sheets on breathing and meditation. We have to realise that if we keep ourselves fit and healthy in body, then the mind has a much better chance too. Then I went swimming, swimming very slowly for 40 minutes. In the afternoon I went to the prayer group meeting at the presbytery for the mental health group. Talking about faces, whose face would we choose to have if we could have a free choice. There was a recent report in the paper about face grafts, and how they can be useful for burns victims, or if someone has had a bad accident or illness. But imagine a choice, now who would I choose to be, young/old/, girl/boy, man/woman/child – very interesting.

In the Library this week I picked up a leaflet called 'Have You Had Manic Depression/Bipolar Disorder?' which is a project by the Institute of Psychiatry, so yesterday I phoned them and said I would be interested in taking part. They wanted to know how many episodes I'd had (2) and if anyone in the family is schizophrenic. Forms for consent arrived today and it all sounds very interesting, so I think I will take part. David checked the form, as it says it also wants family members to take part, if they agree. I'll do this tomorrow.

Saturday 30th November
I just thought it's St Andrews Day – the feast of the Scottish saint. It reminded me of when we were at school in Scotland, and we had white dresses on, with a tartan sash. Now we were entitled to wear the Scottish tartan Lamont which is a green base. Of course the Scottish clans were not catholic, at least I don't see how they could be, because they were so particular about entitlement as to who could wear what. The Campbells and the McDonalds were always fighting – the Glencoe

story is their story. I remember once we went to Glencoe and took the cousins with us, where we saw the Glencoe mountains and the display on the area. Then, on the journey back we all listened to the music tape with the Glencoe story and the wee woman song. It was quite fun, and I remember that we all liked the song, and joined in it together. Another time we took the cousins with us on a 10 day trip to Holland, and met up with their grandma and grandpa in Amsterdam. What fun! Staying in the youth hostels in the family rooms was fun too. Castle Domburg was a big old building with a moat round it, but so near the sea, and we could walk through the castle grounds to get to the sea. We went on a cycle ride on a very windy day, and had to battle to get through.

Footprints is an anon poem and here are those meaningful words:-

'One night a man had a dream. He dreamed he was walking along the beach with the Lord.
Across the sky flashed scenes from his life. For each scene, he noticed
Two sets of footprints in the sand, one belonged to him and the other to the LORD.

When the last scene of his life flashed before him, he looked back
At the footprints in the sand. He noticed that many times along the path of his life
There was only one set of footprints. He also noticed that it happened
At the very lowest and saddest times in his life.

*This really bothered him and he questioned the Lord
about it.*
*LORD, you said that once I decided to follow you,
you'd walk with me all the way.*
*But I have noticed that during the most troublesome
times in my life,*
There is only one set of footprints.
*I don't understand why when I needed you most you
would leave me.*

*The LORD replied, "My precious, precious child, I love
you and I would never leave you.*
*During your times of trial and suffering when you see
only one set of footprints,*
It was then that I carried you." '

There is a game called scissors/paper/stone. Scissors
blunt, paper cuts, stone remains. Can I see you? Can
you feel that? Can I see a voice, or hear a picture?
What happens when our senses get mixed up – they
combine to give strange effects. Like optical illusions,
like hearing voices, or seeing things, or visual
distortions, or strange smells. Space and time are in
different dimensions. They intersect at a point, in space
and in time.

Tuesday 17th December
As a school governor I attended the primary school
Christmas play this afternoon. The children played
bells. There was lots of singing and action round Santa
Claus and his sleigh.

Tuesday 18th February

Just finishing my notes in this book. Breaking the cycle of abuse.

I've been on Rispiredone again (3rd time – 2nd most – 1st was in 1997/98 I think) since 04 February. One at night and morning and then increased to 2x2mg at night over a week and a half ago. It makes me feel quite agitated, as opposed to anxious. I find it difficult to write/to read/to relax. I feel <u>agitated</u>. Agitation is worse than anxiety I feel because you cannot settle. In a queue it is very difficult – I do not like to wait in a Q – I get restless and feel as though I cannot wait, but I have to. My writing is much worse – just compare – I have very little control of the motor function for writing, which makes it (1) harder, (2) less tidy and (3) more difficult to read, so (4) I do not want to write much. So we get to the point where I do not want to sit, stand, write, read, etc.., and consequently my limited attention suffers and in output and input is greatly reduced. I read therefore to ensure that the time I have is put to good use. I felt like doing a picture this afternoon, so got out the paint brush and after drawing some whirls started painting the pink page. I stuck it in my exercise book with a picture of a screaming woman on a boat on the high seas, holding her hands to her ears. Then I compared the two. My picture showed more eyes, more sight, and the face showed a smile, with feelings of terror in the mind. Therefore I concluded my picture was a very internal picture compared with the screaming woman I stuck in. She looks terrified and is saying help me, whereas my picture is saying where am I? A question is a good answer to a question, just another technique in communication skills. I'm not sure I know what U mean. I see it in a different way. Have U thought about?

Being on Rispiredone is a cumulative drug. It feels like more of a knock-on and knock out effect. It makes me increasingly feel tired and listless. It may be helping my brain – hope so, but it makes my body tired. I feel I have to make more and more effort to (1) just get up and (2) to do anything and (3) keep concentration. Today I need to phone up about the NLP, neuron-linguistic psychotherapy I have heard about and see if there is a course for me. I need to explore options for me – what would work and how can I seek help. You only know what's around if someone tells you – it is not advertised at all. Also I do not want a course where some people like to gas and talk about all the options and personal saga. I think some people do not keep things confidential. Read an interesting article in yesterday's Guardian about bereavement. See also the special leaflet on bereavement I picked up at the Mental Health Team offices, and also the 'Change Your Mindset' leaflet issued by MIND, and their other ones on Understanding Depression and Understanding Manic Depression. Manic depression means peaks and troughs, mountains and valleys, highs and lows. But it is OK when you get used to it. Learn to go with the flow in the sense of when it's positive go with it, and when it's negative have a little rest.

Bereavement is a complex state, with feelings and depression, and anger and fear and mixed feelings and also memories of other losses. Note also the links between other losses, like after miscarriage, and feelings associated with post natal depression. Miscarriage is a loss too, miscarriage links in to child protection and child death, like cot deaths, and protecting children and the development of their immune system.

Saturday 22nd February

Rented 3 films, including Bambi which I really wanted to see. Overlaying is an interesting concept in psychiatric conditions. Talented/desperate is that what we are? - going through the gamut of feelings of fear/embarrassment. Choices. Why? Possession – personal or object? Fright? What is all this? I've been on Prozac since 1996/7 after New Year I think. What a long time/term! Protection means needing help too! Remember things. Who are you with. Strength to protect yourself/strength to let go. Only way to help yourself is to go back. Back to that time. Leave him/her alone – need protection – is it too late – who can we protect now? Feelings of being scared/frightened/tearful. Acknowledge those feelings and the name of who someone is. Relate feelings (yours) to other person's feelings. Reverse/inverse feelings like e.g. Mummy/child/child/Mummy. Watching one of my videos, 'Don't Say A Word' I was busy for two hours doing an abstract mind map at the same time. I extrapolated the information from the film and put it into words and pictures in my book.

Monday 24th February

I'm watching and listening to 'Bambi' – lovely songs and words to music – like words and pictures – sing-along time songs for Disney films. I first saw this as a girl I remember with my mum and sisters. Today I got some information on MIND, including the small leaflet on prescriptions and about the new Mental Health legislation – I must read this and try and give some input to this and other campaigns. Bambi seems to be about mothers bringing up their children and absent fathers. The great stag is the great prince of the forest and 'men' is the enemy. Perhaps this is one of the first real environmental films, and gets its message across about the seasons. Bambi's mother was shot, but before she goes she says 'don't look back'. Then the 'great prince' explains Mum can't be with 'Bambi' anymore. So Bambi goes on and grows up. It turns into rather a 'Lion King' story of the cycle of life.

Wednesday 26th February

Today I feel tired. These Rispiredone are cumulative and build up in my body. It's hard sometimes to get up let alone carry on each day. I need to hear from (1) MIND, (2) NGC, (3) Local meeting of the Governor's Council in Camden for the London Governors, (4) local governors council – do they want us to go to conferences or not? Trying hard to eat 5 bits of fruit and veg a day, at least. I wish I could read and write properly – I'm tired.

Thursday 27th February
Met up at the church today and went on our mystery tour to the countryside. Stopped first for morning coffee, then on to a little village for lunch. Had a glass of wine in the pub. Then just to finish off the day in

style after a little walk we had a cream tea. What a mystery tour! Returned home by 6.00 pm.

1st March

Today David and I are going to the theatre to see the Roy Orbison story. I made a shepherd's pie after going shopping with David. I cut out one of the pictures on hearing voices, about schizophrenia, about what the subject feels and hears. I thought it was a very good pictorial representation of something that is <u>not visual</u> as such, but is <u>auditory</u>. Another interesting article in the paper today is an item about sign language for babies and their carers – to increase early communication. Specific useful signs for babies and their early communication needs are 'more', 'pain', 'I love you' and 'milk'.

Monday 3rd March

Today I received a letter from my psychiatrist confirming my medication and that I had presented normally and to be seen again this Friday. 'Her mood is improving and there is no evidence of psychotic illness. Her behaviour during the consultation is much more appropriate.'

Tuesday 4th March

Reading the OHE (Office of Health Economics) booklet on depression and it is quite interesting, especially the photograph on the front of a woman sitting at her living room table with all the cares of the world round about her face. It talks about the iceberg of depression, that is the large amount of depression which is present in the population but still unrecognised by doctors, and it mentions only one quarter are recognised. There are many depressed patients who do not seek medical help for their depression. Some may not know they are depressed and others may be too ashamed. Bipolar depression – manic depressive psychosis occurs with an incidence of 0.5%-2% of the population.

Wednesday 5th March
Preparing this morning for my afternoon meeting concerning children who are excluded from school. Inclusion is the theme.

8th March
Our details on the Marrakech holiday arrived. We are going with David's parents, so posted on a copy to them of the arrangements.

Sunday 16th March
Finished putting the special educational needs ideas together into a report for a policy to send to the school exclusions unit. Really enjoyed this work.

Monday 17th March
Today it's St Patrick's Day and is the end of all the building works in the house for the new bathroom. Hooray!! … Stuck in an article about recovering addicts – the picture of chairs ready for a heart shaped meeting shows the caption, 'Recovering addicts are already in a relationship with a substance. Starting a personal relationship is merely substituting one mood-altering agent for another.

19th March

I go to work at Crimestoppers today. It is interesting how many volunteers they have now and there's always new volunteers presenting. I still feel tired, but I suppose that's not surprising because taking Risperidone in the evening is hard work to get over and through. I think I am doing quite well getting up when I do and getting ready for work, but on the other hand, I feel so much better when I am up and doing – I feel alive and that is vital. I was very worried about the money when I had to keep the business going and also now, because having the two children still around makes life still expensive. I would like to be able to get a job – I don't think I could cope with full time work, but definitely part-time, so that I can earn some money. As I'm working 2 days (almost) a week at the moment, then I should be able to cope with that, or something like that. Dear God please help me to boost up my actions. It's evening time now and after I came home I had to have a little rest. I'd like to copy out some poetry, so here goes on a teacher on teaching practice after qualifying, …

Thursday 20th March

It's another beautiful day. War in Iraq today – prayed for peace at the prayer group meeting.

Friday 21st March

Spent the day from 9-3.30 pm on a Service Users Consultative Forum. Interesting models for development here – use medical and social care model for the joint health and social care course and students. Speech mentioned the manic depression study, so I volunteered information about that and that I had taken part.

I need to earn some money. Can I? David says I should not ghettoise myself – so I need to try and sharpen up. God please help me and David in trying to get ourselves sorted out. Dear God please also help my son to be able to get a job he likes. Also please help my daughter to do well with her studies and to arrange her summer work in America.

Saturday 22nd March
We got up about 9 ish, and today David did not have to go to his course, so we had time at home together. Please dear God help me to be able to get myself organised enough to do things that have to be done. I have put on a wash. I got a letter from the psychiatrist, which I replied to by email. In the afternoon we went for a walk to the National Trust park, and had a cup of tea there. Later David went out to buy some books on Marrakech for our holiday – we set off on Wednesday. In the evening we went to the theatre to see La Traviata – the fallen woman. This Italian opera had subtitles in green, and it was professionally done – excellent. We rounded off the evening by a light meal nearby with a bottle of house wine.

Sunday 23rd March
After yoga and swimming as usual on a Sunday, I wrote in my journal again. A heart with you and me. Where are you says a voice. Me pipes up another. I know where you are coming from – do you care?

Do you know who I am in speech bubbles, and the answer is immediate yes. Then to finish is a picture of peace with the tree of life. Watched a good programme on Buddhism and Nirvana.

Monday 24th March
Today I need to get things ready for our holiday, as tomorrow I go to work then on to the school governor meeting. As I understand it nobody seems to understand manic depression, so it would be good if I could contribute more to the understanding of it by writing a book. The researcher at the Institute of Psychiatry had thanked me after the study interview, because I had said quite a lot. I do remember that I had to keep asking for the question to be repeated when I was on the tape – the bit relating to the past. I did enjoy taking part in the research about me. Perhaps it will benefit me someday too, anyway other people down the line. If I was to write a book which I may, then I'd want to have a catching title like
'They Call Me Manic - It Rhymes With Panic'. Yes I'm manic, maybe you'd be too if you'd been in the Titanic. Manic/Panic/Titanic Bipolar/Stellar/Cellular Disorder/Chaos/Mayhem ,Affective is a word(ld) apart Detached/Spaced out/Apart
'The Chaotic World of My Head'. The world inside my head – so different from the chaos around me, or is it the inverse. I like the poem which Beating Drum sent by post. It goes:

'On Being Yourself'

'You must remember (learn) that you may (can) not be loved by all people.

You may be the finest apple in the world – ripe, juicy, sweet, succulent and offer yourself to all.

But you must remember that there will be people who do not like apples.

You must understand that if you are the world's finest apple, and someone you love does not like apples, you have a choice of becoming a banana.

But you must be warned that if you choose to become a banana, you will be a second-rate banana,.

But you will always be the finest apple.

You must also realise that if you choose to be a second rate banana, there will be people who do not like bananas.

Furthermore, you can spend your life trying to become the best banana – which is impossible if you are an apple – or you can seek again to become the finest apple.'

I wonder if this equally applies to vegetables, as fruit. Because David always said he would look after me even if I was a vegetable. At the time I thought that was sweet, but nothing more. As the years have gone on I like being looked after, and maybe I am a vegetable. What a silly thought!!

'They Call Me Manic – A World of Chaos and Panic'
'A Story of a Mother with Bipolar Affective Disorder'

A Woman Named Peace (from the Circles of Peace winter 1997/98 Newsletter – Universal World Harmony Through Service – May Peace Prevail on Earth.
From 1953 to 98, a remarkable woman who wished to be known simply as 'Peace Pilgrim', walked more than 25,000 miles throughout the United States and Canada on a journey of love. She wished that every person on the planet might experience a bit of the inner peace she felt. She also desired global peace and vowed to continue walking 'remaining a wanderer until mankind has learned the way of peace'.

Traditionally a pilgrimage is a journey of prayer and faith undertaken on foot, and during which time the pilgrim contacts others with a message of hope and love. Wearing a tunic with the words 'Peace Pilgrim' on the front and '25,000 Miles For Peace' on the back, this unique woman encountered many opportunities to speak with others about that mission.

For 8 years Peace Pilgrim offered words of inspiration, coupled with practical suggestions, to those seeking inner peace. 'Never feel sorry for yourself' she admonished. 'Recognise problems as opportunities for growth. Try making a list of the things you have to be thankful for.' She advised that every encounter with another person is an opportunity to 'think of some encouraging thing to say, some good thing to bring – a considerate attitude, a helping hand'.

As word of her peace mission spread, Peace was extensively invited to speak on radio and television or to appear before school, church or community groups.

She used these opportunities to suggest ways to bring about global peace. 'Put the welfare of the whole human family above the welfare of any group,' she advised. 'Have as your objective, the resolving of the conflict, not the gaining of advantage.' She firmly believed that individuals must give up their fears, the greatest 'block to world peace', and told people to 'fear nothing and radiate love'.

Finally, Peace Pilgrim encouraged everyone she met to continue in some way, no matter how small, the work she had begun. 'A few dedicated people can affect the ill effects of masses of out-of-harmony people,' she said. 'Continue to pray for peace and to act for peace. Speak for peace. Live the way of peace. Think of peace and know it is possible. What we dwell upon,' explained Peace Pilgrim, 'we help to bring into manifestation. One little person giving all of her time to peace makes news. Many people giving some of their time can make history.' Friends of Peace Pilgrim, 43480 Cedar Avenue, Hamet, CA 92544 USA – ask for a free copy of 'Steps to Inner Peace'.

Friday 4th April

I have read all my post and emails received while away on holiday, so that brings me up to date. I wish that I could get myself a decent job, say 5 mornings a week – that would be enough to get me going each day and encourage me to develop my abilities. I do have a lot of talents, and really I need a job where these can be showed off and me receive feedback for what I do. Everyone needs to feel valued, and at the moment I need to put out my feelers and get feedback. I do want to be able to establish myself again, and work at Crimestoppers has helped me in this pursuit, but there is so much further to go. David always promised me he would look after me even if I was a vegetable, and it would appear that I have been one of those for a while. But I want to be fresh and alive, not an old lack-lustre type, so I need to get myself going and ensure that I wake up and act like I am alive and have a brain, not be just in a vegetative state. This can be quite hard if you suffer from anxiety – jelly legs and palpitations, etc. When I was at the psychiatrist's office last time I picked up this leaflet on 'Increased Appetite and how to deal with it', along with one on anxiety and what it is by MIND. That was most interesting, and talked about palpitations and jelly legs and panic attacks, so I found it reassuring to hear of other people also experiencing dry mouth and jelly, floppy legs. It can be a learned experience, so we need to learn ways out of it too. On the question of appetite the leaflet suggested that some people find that the medication they are on leads to an increased appetite. It dealt with food cravings, and thinking about our appetites, so that we do not eat to excess and then store this as fat, and it suggested keeping a food diary for a few days. The back page gave some useful tips on keeping your appetite under control. It suggested cutting down on snacks between meals, having a glass of water before and during meals, helping to fill us up without adding any calories, including fruit and vegetables in the diet, as they are filling and also low on calories, limiting the amount of fat in the diet, and trying to keep busy. Sometimes eating is just something to do, so it suggested trying to work out something interesting to do instead, and making a plan of what you will eat and when, then rewarding yourself when you stick to it. I think these points just reinforce what I already know, but it is a bit of a comfort to me to know also that other people experience weight gain on medication like myself. So it is something we need to work on.

The confidence building and self awareness course I did last term was 10 weeks long, and covered the following topics:

Week 1 – objectives for the course and who everyone is.

Week 2 – personal barriers – effective use of time.

Week 3 – personal strengths/development areas/priorities. Effect of increased confidence in their lives.

Week 4 – Awareness of the effect of emotions, and technique for relaxation.

Week 5 – personal influences/reactions to authority and power. Techniques for personal power.

Week 6 – self-awareness on how we give away our own power. Labels – how we got them and what we want to change.

Week 7 – how we build and erode self-esteem and a technique for increasing confidence.

Week 8 – to be aware of the importance of self-love. How we build/erode self esteem.

Week 9 – power of positive thinking, and aspects of confidence.

Week 10 – roundup.

Saturday 5th April

I have just started to read Louise L Hay's book 'You Can Heal Your Life'. I think I'll write down a few useful quotes to keep and think further about. 'If I am willing to affirm for myself that 'Love is everywhere and I am loving and lovable' and to hold on to this affirmation, then it will become true for me. Now, loving people will come into my life and people already in my life will become more loving towards me, and I will find myself easily expressing love to others.

'When we grow up we have a tendency to recreate the emotional involvement of our early home life.' This is what we know as home. 'The point of power is always in the present moment.' What is important in this moment is what you are choosing to think and believe and saw right now. For these thoughts and words will create your future. Do you want this thought to be creating your future? Notice it. Our experiences are just outer effects of inner thoughts. Thoughts can be changed. Change the thought, and the feeling must go. We can change our attitude towards the past, and to release the past we must be willing to forgive.' Louise finds that resentment, criticism, guilt and fear cause more problems than anything else. When we are in a state of panic, it is very difficult to focus our minds on the healing work. We have to take time out to dissolve the fears first. 'I forgive you and I set you free', this affirmation sets us free. All this dis-ease comes from a state of unforgiveness she says. Love thyself. People who love themselves and their bodies neither abuse themselves nor others. It can even enable your body weight to normalise. Criticism locks us into the very pattern we are trying to change. The 'problem is rarely the real problem – when we feel frightened or insecure or not good enough, many of us put on weight for protection. Diets don't work.

Saturday 6th April

'Tomorrow do your worst, for I have lived today.'
It's Joanie's birthday today, so yesterday evening we went over to her house, had a chat, then took her out for a drink. Then we went for a meal of pancakes and vegetables, sizzling prawns and fried rice, followed by banana fritter. Um. David says we have to provide for tomorrow but not live for tomorrow. This is like enjoy the day, which can be fun, or hard work, but whatever, it's movement and progress after involvement in today. It is important to understand this concept, so as not to get too worried or obsessed about anxiety and depression. 'Until someone can show you the connection between the outer experiences and the inner thoughts, you remain a victim in life', says Louise Hay. She shows us a list of problems and their underlying beliefs.

Problem Belief Financial disaster
I am not worthy of having money
No friends -Nobody loves me
Problems with work - I'm not good enough
Always pleasing others - I never get my way

Whatever the problem is, it comes from a thought pattern, and these thought patterns can be changed! 'You are the power in your world! You get to have whatever you choose to think!' According to Louise Hay I need to change myself, not wait for others to change. She goes on to talk about the willingness to release the need for something, and says that when the need is gone, the desire goes. In this way I can release my desire for … fattening foods, excess sleep, laziness, lethargy, wanting to do nothing, resistance to change, etc. She suggests we 'gently untangle that ball of wool of mental knots, just like a ball of wool. Self worth opens many doors she says and reminds us that the way we were treated when we were very little is usually the way we treat ourselves now. So, the same person you are scolding is a 3 year old child within you. Be kind and comfort your inner child she says. Begin to love and approve of yourself, as that's what the little child needs in order to express himself/herself at its highest potential. I am the power in my world. Today is a wonderful day. I choose to make it so. All is well in my world. She says, 'Control the mind and learn how forgiveness of self and others releases us. Your mind is a tool, you can choose to use any way you wish. You are in control of your mind. You use your mind. You can stop thinking those old thoughts. Have this conversation with your mind. Acknowledge that you are in control and what you say goes.

Noel Coward said, 'Nothing is so potent as music.' Music research helps us understand the benefits of music. It related to left and right brain function – perhaps it helps to link together the two brain functions and 'enable' people to relate better. Maybe that is why music has helped benefit people with Alzheimer's. It encourages I believe positive thought and positive action, particularly if people join in, and sing or play an instrument.

Tuesday 8th April

'I am learning to make today a pleasure to experience.'
I approve of myself – say it every day lots of times.
Remember planting seeds and that a seed will grow into
a plant. Remember the seed that didn't want to grow?
Well it's grown now. Think of the positive
affirmations. I experience love wherever I go. I am in
the process of positive changes. I am willing to release
the pattern in me that created these conditions. Just as a
plant grows so too we can demonstrate our desires.

Wednesday 9th April

Had a very good day today. Worked 10 until 3.45
doing a mail shot. Then at 4.30 had a school
governor's meeting, which lasted until 5.30. Then I
bought the shopping for dinner, and then cooked up
mince and potatoes, whilst David made the starter.
Today also I arranged to take part in the pilot project
for consulting older housebound people about the
services they received and would like to receive. The
ad said, 'We are looking for volunteers to find out the
views of older people by interviewing them in their
own homes. Out of pocket expenses will be covered.
As a volunteer you will need to:-
Be an experienced volunteer, attached to an
organisation
Have a genuine interest in older people
Be objective
Have references (preferably a Criminal Records
Bureau)
Be available for training on 10th April 9.30-1.30
Be able to interview 5-10 people during April to May.'

!0th April

Today attended the Volunteer Bureau training on older people. Should be interesting. In the afternoon attended the prayer group meeting again. Tonight watching a TV programme about the Iraqi war. God help us all!!!

Friday 11th April

There is a very useful table of holistic healing recommendations in Louise Hay's book. She deals with body, mind and spirit, and recommends books, therapies, groups, relaxation, exercise, spiritual group work etc. Of course it is American but we would find similar organisations in the UK now increasingly.

1.   Body

Nutrition: Diet, food combining, macrobiotic, natural herbs, vitamins, Bach Flower remedies, homeopathy
Exercise: Yoga, trampoline, walking, dance, cycling, Tai-Chi, martial arts, swimming, sports, etc.
Alternative Therapies: Acupuncture acupressure, colon therapy, reflexology, radionics, chromotherapy, massage and body work, Alexander, bioenergenics, touch for health, deep tissue work, Rolfing, polarity, trager, Reiki.
Relaxation Techniques: Systematic desensitisation, deep breathing, biofeedback, sauna, water therapy (hot tub), slant board, music.
Books: How to get well by Airola; Food is your best medicine by Bieler; Love your body by Hay; Herbally yours by Royal; Getting well again by Simonton

2.   Mind

Affirmations, mental imagery, guided imagery, meditation, loving the self.

Psychological Techniques: Gestalt, hypnosis, NLP, focussing, TA, rebirthing, dream work, psychodrama, past life regression, Jung, humanistic psychotherapies, astrology, art therapy.

Groups: Insight, loving relationships training, ARAS, Ken Keyes groups, all 12-step programmes, aids project, rebirthing.

Books: Visualisation by Bry; The power of affirmations by Fankhauser; Creative visualisation by Gawain; Focusing by Gendlin; Money love by Gilles; Heal your body by Hay; Love is letting go of fear by Jampolsky; Teach only love by Jampolsky; A conscious person's guide to relationships by Keyes; Superbeings by Price; Celebration of breath by Ray; Loving relationships by Ray.

3.   Spirit

Asking for what you want, forgiveness, receiving (allowing the presence of God to enter), accepting, surrendering.

Spiritual Group Work: MSIA, TM, Siddah Foundation, self-realization, religious science, unity.

Books: Your needs met by Addington; Ageless body, timeless mind by Chopra; Real magic by Dyer; Any book by Emmett Fox; Course in miracles by Foundation for Inner Peace; The science of mind by Holmes; The mutant message by Morgan; The manifestation process by Price; The Celestine prophecy by Redfield; The nature of personal reality by Roberts; Autobiography of a Yogi by Yogananda.

Monday 14th April

'Emotional Confidence' by Gael Lindenfield lists an emotional healing strategy in 7 steps, which are,

1. Exploration 2. Expression 3. Comfort 4. Compensation 5. Perspective 6. Channelling 7. Forgiveness. Then I detail the information she gives but I will not reproduce it here now.

Tuesday 15th April

Yesterday I attended the support group for volunteers at the volunteer bureau. It is a joint project between the bureau and MIND. The group is for volunteers with personal experience of mental health issues to share ideas and discuss any particular difficulties it may throw up at the volunteer's place of work. People on their own have a much more difficult time than me, and have to cope alone with all sorts of things. I am in a privileged position. I'm reading more about emotional confidence and then I will want to read the book about self-esteem. I also looked up bi-polar affective disorder on the internet, and there are many, many references which I can research. I would like to put in definitions of manic depression, and also how to manage mood swings and disorders. There are self---help groups and also information about the condition, so a broad range area to study. Nelson Mandela said at his inaugural address in 1994 – 'It's our light not our darkness which frightens us … playing small does not serve the world … we are all meant to shine as children do … as we let our light shine we unconsciously give other people permission to do the same.' Another Mandela quote, 'I felt fear myself more times than I can remember, but I hid it under a mask of boldness. The brave man is not he who does not feel afraid, but he who conquers that fear.'

Wednesday 16th April

I went in to work today and was busy doing internet research again for the forthcoming dinner. It was quite interesting and certainly made the time go quite fast today. It just goes to prove that if there is just even a little brain activity then that generates more interest and motivation. I searched the net on bi-polar affective disorder this evening for 1 hour. I wish there was a cure for mental illness. It seems to be a real ongoing problem. People understand so much about them, but no one can cure them.

Thursday 17th April

Today is Maundy Thursday and the Queen is distributing Maundy money in Gloucestershire. I read about re-evaluation counselling in a co-counselling sort of way, as a radical alternative to psychiatric treatment. Dear God help me to live honestly and decently and to be able to cope with my depression. Sometimes now it feels like a real burden. It did not seem so before, when I was just on Prozac, but since I have had psychotic episodes and am on risperidone, it has been harder. There have been times before when I would cry out in pain, not really knowing that this was an illness, but just wondering whether this was me. Who am I? God made me to know him, love him and serve him in this world and to be happy with him for ever in the next. John Lennon sang the songs, 'Imagine', 'Mind Games' and 'Power to the People' – all of these works are very pertinent now to our lives, what with the Iraqi war and the changes going on in the world.

My Bi-Polar Affective Disorder

Sometimes I do not know why I am feeling sad – it is just a feeling that comes over me, this despite the fact that the weather is lovely, brilliant and warm and sunny, and there is to look forward to the weekend with the holiday, and yet still there is a heaviness. Is it I wonder a bit like an albatross, something that is hanging there round my neck, because it is not yet discharged emotion. Would it be a good idea to say hello to all these emotions and try and discharge them, a bit like wallowing in them as Gael Lindenfield's book suggests. Because then if they have been acknowledged and indulged they can then be discharged, so that the coast is clear. In other words, when those same feelings are encountered again in the future, through a different set of circumstances, then the response is appropriate to that particular set of circumstances and not to all the baggage of the past.
We need to move on from hurtful feelings:-
Illness and death of mother
Attitude of father to family life
Responsibility as oldest daughter in the family
Freedom – personal
Choice to select a partner
Responsibilities of family life
Worries of business life and finances
Worries of family life
Illness of depression varying nature.

Control over condition by education, experience and effort (three ee's!!!)
Future – writing a book as part of the education and self education process, leading to control.
New dawn – new life free from the same lived experiences and emotions that were made in my childhood, because I have <u>learned</u>! So it is important to share with others what it is I have learned, and how I can try and help others with my experiences. This also helps me as it is an aspect of education, which means 'opening up' – educare.

Mental Health

<u>Conventional help/education</u>   <u>alternatives self</u>

Trusted   MIND
Psychiatric treatment   National
Association of Mental Health
Psychiatrists and medication   Therapies like
psychologist, talking therapies
Talking Therapies
        Alternative/complementary therapies
Young and older people   Parallel to
different age groups

            Building blocks to mental health are
            Trust, faith, hope and charity
            Self-awareness and self
            Self-help and therapies
            Work – paid and voluntary
            Emotional health
            Self-esteem and confidence

They say manic depression is likely to have a genetic component. But equally, it can be our experiences, so my experiences as a child, where I was a responsible carer type, influenced my development, and make-up, which then came into play later. That is why I always try and say to the children that they can go on and do what they can do – not be limited by experiences, or any knowledge of past family background. Look at those people who make good – just look at them. We can all do it. People do not all automatically like either apples or bananas, and we may be an apple or a banana or a plum, or a tomato, which is also a fruit, so there you go! On you go – just do it, which was one of my famous phrases in the 80's I think.

Here are some pointers as to the distinctions between mental distress and mental illness

Mental distress
        Mental illness
Upset, worry, problems, causing distress
        unwell? Or well?
Non-medical, emotional, vulnerable, liable to relapse
        Normal or needing

        Treatment?---
Helpful to have a name to the distress Medical model and Definition Value of person Psychiatrists and diagnosis and labels Person Patient

Saturday 19th April

I wanted to read then write out the pattern of positive self-esteem.

High self-esteem experience from Gael Lindenfield:-

I form a belief, either consciously or subconsciously that I am an OK human being

I begin to feel pleasant physical sensations of warmth, relaxation and vitality

In my mind I make specific appreciations about my value, e.g. I look attractive, I am strong, I am clever

I form positive value judgements and beliefs about myself and my potential e.g. I deserve to be happy and have my needs met, to be liked and loved by other people

I experience a sense of increased confidence and optimism

I feel a sense of trust in the world and people round me

I form the belief that the world can and is highly unlikely to be able to meet my needs and wants

I feel the energy levels in my body beginning to rise

I experience my mind becoming more lively and beginning to fill with ideas

I begin to take positive action to get my needs and wants met

I feel a sense of pride and satisfaction and happiness as I experience my needs and wants being met

I form the belief that I have the power to make myself happy and successful whenever I choose to do so

I begin to feel my mind working creatively on ways to overcome any challenging obstacles which stand in my way on my path to success and happiness

I feel my body energized by the excitement of this challenge
I get into action again
I judge my actions to be successful
And then I begin to experience even more forcibly the self-esteem happening all over again … and again!

Tuesday 22nd April

Yesterday on Bank Holiday Monday David and I went out for the day to walk, had lovely lunch in the Bell Inn, and continued walking so had afternoon tea in the tearoom. It was quite tiring but good for us. When we got home David did gardening and I made the dinner. Today I went to see my psychiatrist at 2.40 pm. He asked me how I was, and I said I thought I was OK, but that I was feeling rather empty and also rather tired and lethargic. I said my thoughts were no longer wondering. He said that he is very pleased that Risperidone is keeping my mind straight and he does not want me to reduce the dose as I suggested. I said I find it depressing to be on so many pills. He said that many people on Prozac have described that empty feeling. I told him I had felt tired all the time I've been on Prozac. He suggested that I now STOP PROZAC. I think he feels that the Risperidone helps my mind and he says that is a very good thing and that I can be well on medication. He said it is not a choice option, for example if I had diabetes it would not be any good to cut out meat – it is the same thing, it is not an option. So I will try it without Prozac. I had already switched my Prozac dose to the afternoon, late after 4 ish, so today will be the first day without taking it. What a relief. This must be very good new for me – to stop taking a medication, it is good. I asked him if I should take anything else like a multi-vitamin or anything, but he said no, just to eat 5 pieces of fruit a day. It has carbohydrate in too which is good. So today is good news day. I am to stop taking Prozac and see him again in 8 weeks time, on 24th June.

Plan

1. To lose some weight. Dr said I was a bit overweight wasn't I?
2. More specifically I think I will try and lose 1 stone in weight.
3. I will drink more water, say 2 pints every morning.
4. I will eat more fruit, say 5 pieces each day, today so far I have eaten 1 Satsuma and 1 pear, and drunk 1 glass of orange so that is three helpings/portions.
5. I will eat less – no eating pies/pasties at lunch time. I will take in fruit and also some herbal drinks so that I cut down on caffeine.
6. I will investigate the herbal drinks and see if there is something I can drink to increase my water intake and to cut down on caffeine.
7. I will eat no chocolate for 1 week, and see how that goes.

How do I feel?

Now that the psychiatrist has suggested I do not take the Prozac it seems like a long overdue and sensible step forward. I agree with it. So, instead of 'feeling empty' because there is this long progression of nothingness, but taking pills, I have something very positive, to reduce my medication. That must be good. Also the 2 books which I ordered have arrived. Bi-Polar Disorder – A Guide For Patients and Families, and also the story of someone's illness. It is important to remember families in all of this too. When I became ill my psychiatrist said to me it is an upset for all of the family too, and that is why it is important to take the medication to make sure I do not relapse, and cause worry for the family. It is important for me to stay on the medication and get well. The second book is 'A Brilliant Madness' by Patty Duke and Gloria Hochmann. There in the introduction are useful words, that when the Dr gave her the diagnosis somehow that meant that her illness made sense. I also remember reading the inspirational story of Dr Jamieson, I think her name is Kate, called 'Touched With Fire' which is about a woman's attempts to come to terms with her manic depression to live with it, and to continue her work as a psychiatrist, which she has done. My psychiatrist seems to think that the Risperidone will help me to keep my mind well. He has faith in medication. I asked him again about the CBT, because I said I feel empty, he said CBT would not change me or make me a better person. He said there is nothing wrong with me – on medication I can be well. Well thank goodness for that. Now I need to understand a bit more background information about the condition, which I will do in these books, and come to terms with it. Then I will be able to make some progress. We are not alone. "I'll bet there aren't too many manic depressives around, who haven't at one time or another abused alcohol or drugs. I think it is our attempt to self-medicate, to suppress the highs and to calm down a little and on the low end to go the rest of the way into oblivion." Page 8 of Patty Duke's book - very interesting. I must say this helps me to make sense of my drinking alcohol in the evenings, but my consumption is really quite moderate, and I certainly do not go into oblivion.

Wednesday 23rd April
We have a mug at home which a good friend gave to my daughter and today I was sitting drinking tea, reading the caption which says, 'Some people think you're cute and sweet, and soft and kind and gentle, my friend I know you're round the bend, and marvellously mental.' Very good. I like that.

Today it was my first day off Prozac and I felt fine. In fact when I returned from work I had energy to sit down and write this. There was no one in the house, only the tumble drier going, so obviously someone had been in. What a lovely peaceful evening, the blossom is drifting down from the trees, which now look quite jaded. Off Prozac I'm wondering if I will start to feel less empty, I hope so. I also hope that I will get energy or be able to free my energy instead of it being trapped along with my other emotions in my body. We need to encourage the balance of the biorhythms. Perhaps it would be a good idea to get some people together to talk about their depression. I do know a few.

Reactive depression is different from a biochemical mood disorder. Chemical depressions mean you can't grieve properly/mourn. Once people begin to feel again, it's a step in the right direction. Manic

depressives during their depressive phase may sleep 9, 10 or 11 hours or they may sleep 8 hours and wake up exhausted. This diagnosis of depression is common – with manic depression it is important to find other markers – physical symptoms – changes in energy levels, in sleep patterns, in the libido, in the appetite. In diagnosing manic depressive illness, questions like:-
Are there thyroid problems in your family?
Who had post-partum depression?
Did anyone in your family try to commit suicide?
Was anyone in the family an alcoholic?
Sometimes manic depressives are so slowed down you can't get anything much out of them until they are treated adequately. While they are depressed they can't remember happy things. Age of onset, inertia, profound motor retardation, mum's post-partum depression, aunt's thyroid, etc., etc. Until diagnosis it was as though he had been moving through life with a grey haze in front of him. 'Until he was treated that's what he thought life was like – a grey haze. That's what was normal for him.' Alcohol which is a depressant, is often the drug of choice for someone who is in a depressed mood. Initially it gives him a lift because it releases inhibitions and blunts psychiatric pain – and does it quickly because it is so rapidly absorbed into the bloodstream. The behaviour of alcoholics often parallels the mood swings of those with manic depressive illness. The initial high of the alcoholic looks a lot like the euphoric stage of bi-polar disorder. The lethargy and inertia that come later match the depressive phase. Fortunately, when the use of alcohol has been mainly to self-medicate depression, successful treatment of the illness often eliminates the

need to drink. These are all excerpts from the Patty Duke book again, written in conjunction with a professional who pulls out the relevant factual information and explains the condition and its effect.

Thursday 24th April
Third day without Prozac. I'm feeling more feeling which is good. Shared a bottle of wine yesterday with David in the evening. I want to get rid of the gout feelings I have in my feet – is it due I wonder to Prozac at all. Also, all the lethargy – is it I wonder. Today going to the riverside with my daughter, so only got to take Risperdal in the evening which is a mercy. Did our shopping then had a coffee together. Afternoon I was at the prayer group meeting. The Gospel reading was about the resurrection, and our faith in life everlasting, which has always been important to me, especially when my mother was dying. 'Peace be with you' is mentioned 350 times in the scriptures, and it is said by God and the angels, and we discussed how it was a bit like people today say stay cool – be at peace.

Poems on Mental Health
✓ Sleuthing
Unceremoniously Dumped
✓ Doctor and Patient
✓ Diagnosis and Self Diagnosis
Stigma
Not wanting to be institutionalised
Depression or mania – Living with manic depression
My Carer
Support in the wider community
Wounds

✓ There's no one to speak to
Journaling
✓ Self-help and survival
User and Carer – user of services, carer of carer
Bipolar Affective Disorder and mental health

Sleuthing
It's an amazing feat – I now have a diagnosis
And I believe it to be correct. I'm reading a book about it to make sure
Because I feel I need to know too.
That this is the way I need to be treated.
But it's taken a long time – is it 18 years?
Just long enough for me to get the vote
After years and years of sorrow and tears
The medical profession has taken me into their confidence
And tried to explain my condition
It's bipolar affective disorder, formerly called manic depression.

A long time ago I read a book on depression after having a baby
As I remember nightmares within days of her birth, which lasted for some two weeks.
I also read a lot about hyperactivity in children, though thinking
Now it would have been better to find out about my sensitivity.
I sleuthed over the years to try and discover more about these feelings.
I occasionally saw a doctor about gynaecological and other women's things.

Then 7 years ago I had what I call a nervous breakdown.
It followed some personal stress factors, but brought unexpected mania.
I was treated for depression with various drugs, like Valium and Risperdal and Prozac and remained on Prozac for almost 7 years with a couple of breaks where I tried to wean myself off drugs.
It did not work for me, I became ill again, and now am on Risperdal.

What I understand now is that I am feeling better and am able to write poetry.
My words are better because I can concentrate. I am getting better.
Psychiatrically it is a success story, so I am relieved.
So is my doctor, that I can get better being on medication.
I have not quite got used to it yet, but I'm trying.
It's far better that I learn to live again, a productive life
To increase my voluntary work to the point where I trust myself
And feel confident enough to seek a paid job.
The task is one 'to do'.
What progress from some 8 months ago when I was just trying 'to be'.
I was desperate and did not know which way to turn, so I was
Invited into a support group in the church
Once a week I had my own group meeting where we prayed together.
I had just had a diagnosis and I felt lost.
Now 3 seasons further on, I have also moved on.

I am learning to be at peace with myself, and return to
A healthy, balanced life. At least I know now.
So I'm hoping to meet plenty of people and talk
To them too, bit by bit, about my experiences.
Sleuthing is hard work. There's lots more to do.

Unceremoniously Dumped

It was when I was vulnerable and feeling lost
No one seemed to be helping me professionally.
I had appointments, then I was left alone.
I no longer saw the psychiatrist and was referred back
to my GP.
I had said I wanted to try and get a job.
Now, I think that was totally unrealistic.
10 months further on, and I'm still not confident
enough to
job search, let alone hold down paid work.
So, somehow I managed to have an appointment with
someone new.
I had been referred to the Occupational Therapist.
I remember waiting day by day for the appointment.
In between times I was at home, resting, feeling tired
and depressed.
So I pinned a lot of hope on this appointment.
I had recently been diagnosed as manic depressive,
But it had not sunk in.
I felt tired and lethargic, but I was not mentally ill.
I was depressed but I was not clinically anything more
than that.
I even came off Risperdal and I felt a wreck.
I had no confidence. I cried so easily. I felt very
sensitive and

Vulnerable, but I did not feel ill.

The day of my appointment arrived and I went to see the OT.

I walked along – 20 minutes to the hospital – it felt like an hour.

I was tired when I got there and agitated and after introducing myself to her I cried.

It was so exhausting being ill and short of words.

Nothing made sense.

Why was I there?

Surely I could get a job without specialist help? But no – I could not.

I remember how I desperately wanted to appear normal.

But it was all too much for me and I cried and felt so sad.

Why was I sitting opposite an OT? And talking about myself?

At least I wasn't talking to myself then.

I agreed to do some voluntary work to get myself on my feet again,

And arranged to go with the OT to the volunteer bureau –

She would make an appointment for us.

So, some 2-3 weeks later she came to my house and took me along for the appointment.

I wouldn't have made it without her, but she thought I seemed fine –

I put on a brave face at first, but then again I cried.

As I was introduced to the volunteer bureau that was my only dealings with the Occupational Therapist.

So again I was dumped, unceremoniously to get on with life on my own again.

There never was anyone to talk to.

There never is anyone to really speak to

Oh help – I need someone to talk to –
Someone who will listen to me, maybe come for a
coffee
Or talk to me slowly about their life too.
Why is there no one there?
I thought there was care in the community?
But there's no care for me – there's no one to talk to.
I need someone to be there for me, just for me, now or
when I feel lonely.
It feels as though I'm alone – deserted on this planet.
The last one left alive here, but what a lonely life.
There's no one to talk to.
There's no one to speak with.
Everyone is busy with their own life, and talking away
On the phone, in the street, in the shops, on the radio
and TV.
But there's no one for me.
No one is here where I am, alone, feeling lonely, but
Unable to really speak up for myself.
I feel lost and withdrawn but want someone to speak to.
O once tried the Samaritans but it's a bit anonymous
over the phone.
I want to see someone and talk to them.
I'd really like to have a voluntary visitor and phoned an
agency who sent round volunteers
But you needed to qualify for their service and I didn't.
So I couldn't have a voluntary visitor.
I'm not elderly or housebound as such, although I often
felt completely trapped
In my own house, afraid to go out.

Then I was sometimes too tired to concentrate for the radio and the TV, and I couldn't read.

I felt tired, but I would have liked a voluntary visitor to speak to.

There never was anyone to speak to.

Friday 25th April
Rejoice the Lord is Risen, Alleluia, Easter!

Do not lose heart, said Werenfried van Straaten, Founder of Aid to the Church In Need. 'The Church is greater than a Professor's Chair in Tubingen, or a handful of prophets and rebel clerics who for the time being hold sway in the media. For she bestrides all the frontiers of the earth and draws her imperishable vitality from the Risen Christ who has said, 'When these things begin to take place, look up and raise your heads, because your redemption is drawing near.''

Message of our Lady of Medjugorje for March.
'Dear children! Also today I call you to pray for peace. Pray with the heart, little children, and do not lose hope because God loves his creatures. He desires to save you, one by one, though my coming here. I call you to the way of holiness. Pray, and in prayer you are open to God's will: in this way, in everything you do, you realise God's plan in you and through you. Thank you for having responded to my call.'

Today I felt rather tired. In the evening as usual on a Friday we went to yoga and swimming. I feel so much better on return from this. Of course maybe it is just relief that I have done the class and that I managed to do it. Because en route I did not feel I would be able to cope. It just goes to show you can have these feelings of not being able to cope and do things, and then you can. Dear God please help me to be able to do more and to feel that I have the energy to do this.

Saturday 26th April

Perhaps I should keep a life chart. This is a day by day chart showing how you feel and helps you to feel in charge of your condition. I wish that I did not have this manic depressive illness. It's really horrid, and so is it that in the end the sympathy runs out. I'm coming off Prozac, and I feel very tearful. I turned to David for sympathy and he tells me that it is an illusion, because of coming off the drug. It is like getting in touch with my feelings again. Where have they been? Hiding away in a dark hole somewhere too difficult to find, or to invite out into the open again. It is very difficult trying to understand that I can 'feel' again. But I'm so scared, I'm so scared. Why is this? Where am I really feeling – is it in my head or in my heart, or in my hands. Yes, it's in my hands. I feel I want to express my feelings, so I take to writing which is a written expression, through my hands. I could also touch people like I try to do. When I rang Joanie yesterday I wanted someone to speak to. There's unfortunately now very few people to speak to, because I just don't have the stamina to make friends any more. Yes, I make contacts with people, and so it is a good idea to come along to gatherings and see how I feel when I am there. And yes I do need to find out some information about manic depression, but I should not dwell on it as Joanie says. I need information and details about the process of depression and mania, but there must be more to it than that.

Rethink, formerly the National Schizophrenia Fellowship is a self help group, and they have local meetings too. They offer advice, information and support for carers and sufferers both at meetings and on the telephone. Speakers include psychiatrists and other mental health professionals, pharmacists and benefits advisers. 'If someone in your family has, or is developing, a serious mental health problem such as schizophrenia or depression, do come along to this friendly self-help group.' I picked this leaflet up at the out patient clinic again last time I was there. Would this be any use for me I wonder.

Sunday 27th April
On Saturday evening David and I went out to see the film, 'Johnny English' which turned out to be very good – quite funny. The Bond type cop managed to do the big things very well, just did silly little things which were amusingly good. The audience enjoyed the film too. Then we tried to go to the Indian restaurant but it was full up, so we headed off to the Chinese one which gave us a nice meal as per usual, and also one of the only places in town to do banana fritters. Today, the Sunday, is a beautiful day. We enjoyed our early morning yoga class and then a swim before coming back to a chicken lunch. Afternoon, the sun shone brilliantly so we headed off for a walk up on the common beside the two lakes, and then a cup of tea in the tearoom. This year we have a little wisteria in bloom – hysterical wisteria. There is a little wisteria

growing along the line of the garage. Laburnam grows also in 2 places – one on either neighbour's fences. As yet only a little bloom of yellow. The keria is coming out – one in a pot, and one in the flower bed. I've got 2 hanging baskets – one with Primulas and the other with pansies. Both are OK and flowering well, after a long dry spell where we had to take them down and water them. The clematis is in bloom ready to display on the dividing boundary trellis between the neighbours and our patio. We share the side and front path with them, which is quite a nuisance having to have a shared path. In all my previous houses I had my own path, so it is a bit of a burden.

Monday 28th April

Today it is raining as predicted by the weather forecast. I must say that my head is feeling clearer, and I am able to concentrate quite well. This is such an improvement, and one to be thankful for. The only thing is that I do not have a job – I would like one of those, so I think I will try and go into the job centre or one of the employment agencies say at the end of the week. It would be an achievement if I could get myself back together, enough to work, even say part-time, to earn some money to support the family home. I feel as though I am not keeping my end up in all this, and I should like to do better. I just need a little job – say part-time that pays OK, so that I can feel as though I am paid, and contributing to the family finances. Also I want to lose weight. I need to get one of those funny skinny fish to stick to the fridge, to remind me that I could be slimmer. Anyway for breakfast I had a yogurt, and also 3 glasses of water, and some coffee. I did not feel particularly hungry so it was no hardship for me. Today I want to read a bit more of the book 'A Brilliant Madness' so that I can finish it soon. Did a little sketch of sunrise on the horizon. I think I will buy some flowers too.

Diagnosis and Self-Diagnosis

Self-diagnosis is a dangerous condition.
I know because I have tried it once for a long time.
It isn't that I wanted to be a doctor, or anything medical.
In fact I am a traditionalist in the sense of believing that doctors are in charge.
However, I like to know what is wrong with me, and to take a positive role in the process.
I used to think it was just depression as did my doctor.
I used to have strange feelings in my head where I imagined fancifully.
I would think that the children were little fish, peeping out from behind a rock to dart in and out of sight.
I wanted to buy those fish at the aquarium and take them home.
I was checked in this behaviour by my relatives who explained about the fish
Being happy in the aquarium and that I could not cope with without an aquarium.
So family are important in the diagnostic and self diagnosis procedure.
We must listen to others or we are in danger of losing touch with reality.

So, today in the post I received a letter from my psychiatrist.

It is a copy of the one he writes to my GP.

It says, "I saw this lady on 22nd April. She is well in herself and her mood is stable.

She complains of feeling lethargic and an inner feeling of emptiness.

We had a long discussion about her medications.

I suggested that it is important that she remain on the Risperidone but the Prozac is less important.

It is the Prozac that may be contributing to the feeling of emptiness which she described and finds distressing.

We therefore agreed that she may remain on the Risperidone at a dose of 4 mg a day, but that she discontinue the Prozac.'

The Psychiatrist emphasises the importance of remaining on the Risperidone in order to prevent further relapses. He has arranged to see me again in 8 weeks time.

This joint approach to diagnosis and treatment is helpful. It makes me feel that I am in charge of my own future too.

I like getting copy letters – it is important to me and my self-esteem.

Also, I find it useful now that I have a diagnosis of bipolar affective disorder to read about this.

I bought 2 books – one written by a doctor for patients and their families with the condition.

And a second, being a collaborative approach by an actress with manic depression and a medical specialist in the field.

They both give me more information which is another important part of management of the condition.

In reading these books, I can identify with some of the feelings and situations expressed in the book.
And this helps me recognise that I am not alone.
Also now that I have a diagnosis, I have the option of joining a self-help group.
In my view it opens the door to further progress, rather than just labelling.
So I have a particular condition, but I am also me, that unique, special human being.
And my family value me in their own particular way,
And together with other support contacts and friends, help me value myself and start looking to the future.

Doctor and Patient

Her behaviour was inappropriate was one of the phrases the Doctor used.
She was paranoid was another.
My psychiatrist writes me copy letters of the reports he sends to my GP about my care.
I'm grateful for these – they provide a link between one appointment and the next, and describe my behaviour.
I find this very useful, as an objective test of who I am, and the way I have presented to the doctor for attention.
Usually I cannot remember who said what, unless I write about it straight after the interview as I sometimes do.
Last time for example we held a discussion about the effects of my medication, and agreed that I would continue on one drug, as prescribed, which I had been getting used to for some 4 or so months, and the other drug I would stop.

251

We discussed, or rather he told me and I heard about the side effects can sometimes make you feel empty and lethargic.

So we decided and agreed I would stop that drug.

I wanted to feel, and I wanted to try and be me again, not some drugged up patient who can't say boo to a goose.

Sometimes I've ended up saying 'Yes Doctor' when I've been given a psychiatric opinion.

I mean I do not know, how can I possibly equal the expertise of a doctor who's studied psychiatry for more years then I've been ill.

I think I know myself but I need that objective assessment of my condition.

It is a very personal relationship this – telling my doctor how I feel and how I've been.

But it's very difficult to describe my feelings, especially if I'm feeling paranoid, or I'm obsessed about some detail of my childhood.

But I try. I've been feeling empty for 7 years Doctor. Why I wonder do I bring this up now, when I've not mentioned it before?

Is it because the other medication I've been on is starting to work and I now am able to collect my thoughts and describe the concentration of feelings? I think so.

Also, I'm getting to know my psychiatrist now, and because the medication is working we seem to have struck a rapport.

He is pleased that I can get better on medication, and I am relieved my thoughts are starting to focus, and to stop wandering around my head.

This reinforces the belief that psychiatry as a model of care can and does work,
So we both feel the Doctor/Patient relationship is worthwhile.
I'm learning through experience to have confidence in my psychiatrist, which is a very important step when we are talking about problems with the mind, which translate to bodily functions.
Let us build on this Doctor Patient relationship.

Tuesday 29th April
 Self-Help and Survival I think this topic naturally follows on from the one of Doctor and patient. I need to talk about the feelings and how much responsibility we hold for our survival – it is not only just dependent on the psychiatric appointments we have. Groups and reading, and trying to impose a regular kind of a discipline. Survival is linked into feelings of out-of-control, and being a victim of circumstance, etc.
Anyway in the meantime, off I go to work today, and also then I have a meeting later about children who are excluded from school.

Wednesday 30th April
Self-Help and Survival

Yes we have a responsibility for our own health, after we have seen our doctor.
The professional opinion is a good starting point for our action.
It grounds us to the medical model, which we may choose to complement or supplement.

Many doctors nowadays believe in self-help and patient care may well include complementary therapy.

We have moved a long way from the paternalistic view where the professional doctor always knows best.

Many people believe in taking a second opinion, and will discuss their care at some length.

The economics of health care are very complicated.

As a patient I appreciate the consultant and GP care I have had.

I have been told about various self-help and educational resources to supplement my care.

These include e.g. counselling sessions and support health groups.

I have taken a counselling course for about 3 months and found that beneficial

In understanding the true position I was in, aside from the medical diagnosis.

It is crucial to really be able to comprehend the all-round situation.

Why is it that I might choose to take this treatment, or follow that course of action?

I need to know what I think about my health and social care.

I need to understand my feelings about my illness, so that I can take up offers of help.

I need to be able to evaluate support groups on offer.

Do I want to meet other people who are in a similar position to myself?

Do I want to share my feelings in a support group for people with a similar diagnosis.

All these are crucial factors to find out about.

I want to do more than survive.

Although sometimes that is the scenario – how can I survive?
Life has to be more than existence on a day to day basis.
So, I need to learn to help myself, to find out what else is on offer, and how that might be just what I need.

Thursday 1st May

Pinch, punch, first of the month – it's the first day of a new month, how time flies. Phoned my friend in the prayer group to remind her about the afternoon session, and said good-bye to my daughter who went back to university today again. Arranged to see her in June, to pick up her belongings she does not need for next year.

Not Wanting To Be Institutionalised

I haven't been admitted to hospital for mental illness, although my doctor did ask me.
I declined the offer, because I did not want to be institutionalised.
I had the freedom of choice.
I did not have to think about it, I just knew.
I did not want to give up the tenuous hold I had on my life at that time,
So I knew it was best to just struggle on.
Life at home was fine, because I knew what was what.
I knew my room, and the activities I could get involved in, and I liked that.
It was safe because it was comforting and comfortable.
So I did not want to go in for observation, or for a rest, I said no.

But many of my friends have been into hospital and some have talked about their experiences.

Yes, for some it was a rest, a security, when they felt unable to cope at home, and it was the right thing to do.

For some, they missed the independence, of being able to go for a walk when they wanted to.

For others, the hospital setting was the regularity that they needed.

It gave the doctor and nurses, their carers, the time to sort out

A change in medication and see how they were coping with this alteration.

It meant that the user could be more closely observed by the carers, and hopefully, therefore get the care he or she needed.

There is always the danger though that the strength of the carers makes you feel safe in itself,

So you want to stay on.

It is easy to get into a routine at the hospital, with regular meals being provided and the day to day existence of the wards and their visitors.

Perhaps, for some, there comes a point where they feel it is easier on the inside, so they want to stay.

This becomes the danger of institutionalisation, especially if there is a difficulty with medication, and stabilising the care needed.

At what point do we decide that the stigma of hospital admission is worth it, and we decide it is necessary?

Of course, there comes a point if the doctor decides that it is essential, then we really have no choice.

It is at this point that the issue of institutionalisation does not really come into the picture at all, because we need the essential care.

So, stigma and institutionalisation are not relevant at the point of admission.

It is just later, when we are getting better that it matters.

Then, that age old problem of society's definition of mental illness comes into play.

Society thinks that if you have a mental illness you are dangerous and need to be inside.

Then, once inside, you are labeled with the definition of institutionalised care.

So, really, as yet, we cannot win, until we decide to talk about our experiences.

We need to speak up and say that mental illness is treatable, and that mental health is the aim.

We may be institutionalised, or not.

We may be able to cope with care in the community.

It's just that we do not want to be stigmatized by society. That's all.

Loneliness and Despair

Loneliness is a three syllable word, but it sounds so sad.

We need to remember the music which goes with the sounds, so we don't feel so bad.

Good lyrics, rhyme and songs always have the power to cheer us up.

And everything is imbued with meaning when we have rare, exposed emotions.

We understand that the words really speak to us.

It's like listening to the radio or television.

We are finely attuned to the meanings of words and phrases.

It's like we really understand the meaning of meanings.

Our heightened awareness carries us through.

Have you ever felt that the words are just for you?

I have, and its' quite a powerful medium.

Imagine getting your message across to someone who is really listening for inspiration.

It's vital to appreciate the feelings of loneliness before you try and get through to us.

It doesn't just mean there's no one to talk to – it's a whole lot more.

It's much deeper and describes an emptiness of the soul within.

It means this is a wake-up call for us all.

We need to understand what it's like to feel lonely.

Imagine that suddenly all your previous life experiences do not count that you are thrown in at the deep end.

To see if you sink or swim.

Now that is loneliness.

Imagine that our previous confidantes and friends no longer seem to comprehend what you are saying.

That you are still speaking up and saying what you think but that your words seem to fall on deaf ears.

I suppose it's a bit like paranoia – aloneness.

Imagine being suddenly alone, not with the luxury of a lovely desert island with palm trees and gently lapping waves,

But say in a dark, damp cave, where the occasional screech of a bat, or the batting of their wings can be heard, but not seen.

Then, imagine being trapped at the bottom of a deep well and unable to see anything or to climb out or up in any way.

Then add time, and it seems like an endless nothingness.

Now perhaps that is loneliness, but it is very difficult if not impossible, to put it into words.

What happens next?

There may be people anxiously peering down that well trying and straining to see something but not able to make any contact whatsoever.

There may be an exit to the cave just round the corner, but you don't know that and there's no light.

So there's help round the bend or above the deep cavern, but there's no way to access it, because we don't know it's there.

Gosh – now that's isolation and loneliness.

Imagine the feelings of loneliness and how that would lead to wondering if you'd ever get out of there ever?

So, is that despair – I think it is.

It's a wonder that we manage to survive despair but we do.

Friday 2nd May

My daughter left yesterday, back to campus life and I felt very sad and emotional to feel alone again. Is it because we were so close as she was growing up, and now, I see her heading off on her own into the sunset? But that is good, so good. We want our children to have fun, and to be independent, that is what we want for them. When we had the children we did not have them to hang on to them for ourselves, we wanted them to be free and to find their own spirits. Dear God help me to appreciate my children, and to let them be free, and to forge their way in society. When I think of other things I have done to try and help children in general it is quite good – I have done quite a bit helping other people. I became a school governor, and have done some work with the unit for children excluded from school. It's a little bit of expertise, so I feel quite privileged to be part of it – there's a lot of expertise within there supporting the children who are there because of school exclusion, or I believe also refusal, where they have special kinds of difficulties and problems. Some have difficulty with the journey to school – I can relate to that. Sometimes I worry about getting along to a meeting in time, I like to leave in plenty of time, so that I can get there to be ready when it starts. Dear God help me to live a decent life – help me to value myself and my contribution to society, or what is going on. Try to live each day. Is death a great adventure? When it's near the end, perhaps we have a feeling of calmness, so that there is no anguish and pain. I remember when I reviewed the book on sorrow and death and grief and I learned a lot about it. Are we surrounded by evidence of death – yes we are in times of war, but it is usually a very glorified image. Real death, quiet and peaceful and spirituality helps us. Yesterday at the prayer group meeting I enjoyed myself. We discussed positive views and images of disability, and how people with disabilities do love a lot of their views being put forward. People can be admired for their own achievements, whether disabled or not.

I heard a programme on the radio about ECT treatment for severe mental illness, as a last resort. MIND has campaigned against this. Voltage levels are important. ECT – swimming in a cave with no air and rock above. ECT for some people is very helpful. Do people know what they are doing? Last resort option. Hospital guidelines and general ECT Guidance. MIND says on new guidelines, they are welcome news. There is a need for proper regulation and administration under the guidelines. Consent? Make wishes known before become ill, choices to make choices before become ill. Is it appropriate treatment for severe depression? Need a national information leaflet. Dear God do help me to try and get myself better. Help me to stop drinking wine which is a depressant. Help me to stop drinking coffee which is a stimulant and caffeine, and help me to drink lots of water as I did in the summer. Help me to get to grips with my treatment and for my psychiatrist to understand me. Off Prozac I've certainly been more emotional . Help me please God.

David phoned and I just burst out crying. I told him I had strange feelings about my father, when my mother died I just did not have any feelings towards my father. He wanted me to meet him sometimes, to go with him to his do's and even sometimes to the theatre. God why do I feel this way towards my father. He still presumes I am, and my sisters too, are his little girl. He helped us pay for the education of our children, which is very helpful. My mother fell ill when she knew that she had to go up to Scotland to live, why? Maybe she just did not want that change. When I was a child I was always smiling, trying to cheer people up and pretend that things were OK, but deep in my heart I felt alone and sad. I did not want things to be the way that they were. My parents did not come to school dos, I wish they would have. It's like being in a throw-back to those times. It's like looking inwards on all those feelings which I submerged at the time, so that I could get on with my life, because otherwise it would have been too emotional. God do I hate or what? I expect my father really wanted the promotion with going to Scotland, and the social prestige etc., whereas my mother got very little. I don't think she particularly liked it, even though she was a Scot too. God, David doesn't realise how lucky he is to have two parents alive into his middle age. He's been very lucky. Whereas it's me who's been the unlucky one I'm afraid. Yet at the time I pretended to everyone I had a happy life and I tried to find out from David why he felt so sad. But maybe it was just an echo of my sadness that I saw. God my job as a social worker was tough. I just wanted to commune with people and find out what made them tick I think. Why oh why did I collapse after my step-mother died? How many times have I felt really torn up inside – and my insides were like falling out. Thank God the change and all that is now behind me, I hate feeling so dependent on my feelings as well. Perhaps I was never really loved by my father in the deepest sense, so it's no surprise that I really chose a life partner who would love me. David has always loved me. Thank God. What a difficult person I am to love I think because I was always the one giving love before, so there was nothing left. That's why God let me have a car accident, so I relaxed and slowed down for a little while, just about the time I met and got involved with David. A bump on the head did me good. I wanted to find my childhood toy, my lamby which my mother had bought for me, and repaired many times as it was so well used. I wanted to cuddle my lamby and remember it as it was. I was so sad. That was my real feeling of all those years ago. There was nothing to smile and laugh about.

Loss	Happiness
Grief	Graduation
Death	Yuck, my mother was dying.
Graduation	Death

I did not want to go to my graduation because I felt terrible. Would you want to? I doubt it. My mother died the next day. Oh God all this time I've been without my mother. All this time. She just hasn't been there at all. It's just not fair is it, it's not fair. But then look at that little boy injured in the Iraqi war so badly, now without arms. He has no arms now that little mite. My grandmother lived to 101 for God's sake. 101 how is that possible when my mother died at 56 – again it's just not fair is it. But what about all those people who die from cancer? It's not my father's fault. He was a victim as everyone else was. Catholics believe in life after death, as do many other faith believers. The pieta is a lovely statue in many churches. It is hell for any mother who has to take her own son down from the cross. Jesus was dead, but later he rose from the tomb, from the dead, and he said, 'Peace be with you'. Dear God, help us all to recover from the ills of life. Now it is Turkey and another earthquake. Dear God help us all. Love is what we need. |'m glad that I am on medication to control my psychotic symptoms. Now I just need to get better. I need to understand my feelings –why I feel angry. Yet all these years the anger came out against my family, my own little family. My poor family had to put up with me - yes with me. I'm just so horrid, sometimes, the little girl who was so horrid sometimes, the little girl who was so horrid or so nice.

In fact I was a good girl, but now being older I want to get back at those feelings which were really of anger – suppressed and repressed, leading to obsessional good behaviour. Yes I was a good girl. Yuck.

Bipolar II is characterised by fully developed depressive episodes and episodes of hypomania. Bipolar II patients seem to have more problems with depression – in fact the depression is so prominent that many receive a diagnosis of depressive disorder and don't get treatment for bipolar disorder at all. Bipolar II patients had longer depressive episodes than Bipolar I patients (52.2 weeks to 24.3 weeks). Bipolar II patients have also found to be at higher risk for alcoholism. Diagnosis takes a long time to be made – often the person is just thought to be depressive. Bipolar II can perhaps best be thought of as a milder form of Bipolar I. It's more common also. Bipolar I is the more complicated and more severe form – perhaps 1 gene for mood disorder. All this information from my book written for patients and families with Bipolar Disorder.

Monday 5th May
<u>My Carer Looking Inward Focus</u>

Let me tell you about my carer. He is a man named David.
He is my husband of 5 years, and friend for 5 years before that.
My carer cares for me by loving me in a tough kind of way.

Not for him the gentle easing, rather the necessary push and pull
Because I am not an easy person to care for.
I demand attention. I need to be cared for.
But it was not always this way and maybe won't always be
I don't know. I hope not.
But for 7 years I have been looked after with care and love.
Before that I felt as though I was the carer, for my
Husband and my two children – definitely a full-time job.
My life centred around providing for their care.
Until I became ill with a multitude of pressures.
Then, I became the cared for, the one who was looked after.
And I have valued that care. He looks after me.
Sometimes we go for a walk and he will encourage me on.
Or to a yoga class and he will say let's go.
Every time I complete a task I feel better.
He also can feel success at my achievement.
Just like a parent is happy at the child's reward for completing a lesson.
He is my teacher, helping me to learn again how to do it.
It may be a walk, or a process of pruning the plants in the garden.
Or getting up, instead of 729 reasons just to stay in bed.
He is there for me to help me and he makes my day.
So day by day we learn.

Focus on looking inward

I like looking in on myself quite a lot.

I wonder who I am, what am I doing here.

It is sort of like a philosophy question, but more than that.

It really involves my mind and the expressions of feelings.

Wednesday 7th May

Journaling

Notes, ideas, thoughts on to paper. Can see something I've done, because can hardly read. Helps to see something constructive. Sorting out thoughts that are all going round the head. Very useful to be able to put them on paper. Expression and exploration of feelings. Instead of just being in the head, makes it more concrete and definite. Often then can read back what I was thinking even earlier in the day. Amazing framework for expression and exploration. Why is started. Why I took to journaling – every day as a routine, not everyday to just write for the sake of it, but to progress my thoughts and feelings and help get them into some kind of order. Disjointed mix of unbounded thoughts in my head, going off in all directions. Helps with a focus to do journaling. Can write about anything I chose to write about – freedom of expression – my thoughts and no controls. Do not have the usual interactions with others when express feeling or emotion, so it is like a safety barrier too. Can come back to explore the thoughts on another day, because have a ready reference, or just use it as a means of communicating – even with myself. Find it best just to think and write myself. Did not follow on conversations day by day, so mine would be rather a disjointed journal to read, others may have a more flowing expression. It depends on your need. I did not write mine to be read by anyone other than myself. Have shown my family, but they have little interest in the day to day writings. Now have 3 books. First one was a pretty, flower diary, small and unlined and would encourage me to write in it. My daughter even left me a message in it. I have told other people of the method and found quite a few who also wanted to journal, some who did and others who had not heard about it. It keeps us in touch with ourselves.

Friday 9th May

Today I went with the prayer group the Thursday group Richmond Park for a walk. We had coffee first then lunch out. It was a very pleasant interlude and we enjoyed ourselves. Then an early home after lunch, so I went for a coffee with my friend at her flat. My son hoovered the house for me today and also cleaned the kitchen utility room floor. I had previously been to the job centre for an 11 o'clock appointment about getting a job. She suggested I apply for Incapacity Benefit, so I was given the form and made an appointment to see my GP.

Monday 12th May

I went to a conference organised and run by UK Education Forum on the topic of school agreements. These were introduced in 1999 for maintained schools. Quite interesting and I later did a one page summary of the day. Made a green salad, and bought lots of fruit. I'd like to read a book at the moment, it's sort of a continuous process, should I read one on the gypsies that I have. I need to read. I wrote 4 postcards this evening. Do I want to sell books to schools, as a self-employed person – I should think about that.

Friday 16th May

Yesterday I sent my daughter an email and she sent me one straight back so it proves communication works. That made me feel good. Went for tea yesterday with a friend after the prayer group – she had made me a sponge cake, especially for me. She encouraged me to get up in the mornings and get on, and we talked about the prayer group meeting. Do not be afraid for I have come to save you, make space in your hearts for me, and I will be there. God our father help us. The prayer group reading was I am the vine and you are the branches. A vine wanders everywhere. God is our leader – God takes us forward. God help me. Please. Having come off Prozac now I do feel better. I feel more open and aware, but what I also feel is flat, rather at a loose end. The Risperdal keeps my head together. It stops my mind wandering off in a different direction – i.e. more than one way at a time. It is a bit like the mind-blowing bit. When the disciples were in an upstairs room, Jesus appeared to them. He said, 'Do not be afraid.' Please God help us all in the group, and in my family. I have a husband and 2 children. Joanie said that she had more to do with my dad now than she did in the past. She thinks he's lonely and rather isolated these days. He seems to be busy travelling around. He sees my sister more because she is more central than me I suppose. Also I expect he feels that they get on better together than with me, because I am rather quieter. I remember one time he came to this house and we sat all day having tea, and then a lunch. He seemed to be speaking a lot but not me. It did not seem to connect with me at all. I suppose that is just the way it was, no real contact with fathers, who had had a busy business life. Why is it I feel I could have been anyone, and that we ended up having no real relationship at all. Dear God help me understand what has been happening to me, and what I have been through. I do not know what else I could have done. But now here I am, as it says in the words of the school RE programme. Here I am, and need to acknowledge where I am, and then see about going forward. I hope that I will be able to cope with life. Repeat prescriptions can cost a lot of money, and also they mean that you do not stay around at the GP's much. You just call in or write for a repeat prescription and the GP produces one. There is no real need to see the GP. God I'm so lonely. So lonely. I feel as though I do not have any friends, and I need to make contact with other people. I do wish there was a prescription for loneliness – that we could meet up with other people. Dear God please help me.

Sunday 18th May
Let us hope that both the children make it in their chosen fields, music and film. They have both had a lot of exposure to the arts over the years, at home, and in their childhoods. I think now that I am off Prozac I am feeling the real feelings. I seem to need Risperdal to keep my head together. Perhaps it is that I do not really

seem to like myself. I need to learn to appreciate myself more, to learn to love myself and to do nice things for myself and to expect nice things to happen. I do like the statue in the church of the Pieta. I remember when I was ill, I liked that model of Mary caring for her son, and I likened myself to her, which seemed to be a religious experience. There are so many religious experiences I had – I felt, as others have felt, that I was in the Holy Family and we had an extra child, a daughter who would save the world. It is not blasphemous, it is just illness. The reason people focus on religious figures and especially the Holy Family is because they are so familiar to us, and we can liken our experiences in some sense to the living holy family and Christ. I am the vine – you are the branches. Christ is the vine and the branches need to be pruned so that they produce good fruit. The bad leaves are cut back to provide for the good new growth of the living plant.

20th May
<u>Just Convalescing</u>

David says I'm just convalescing – I don't know
I've been unwell for so long, it becomes a way of life.
That's why it's so important to have a standard to live up to
And I mean to grow towards it.
I intend to make progress towards my goal of independence.
At present and over the last few months I have had so many ups and downs – it's like a roller-coaster.
One minute I'm OK, the next I'll be dissolving in tears in temporary despair.

Of course now it could be cold turkey – coming off
Prozac, which I've been doing for the last 4 weeks.
It's not so severe as last summer, when I was on Prozac
and came off Risperdal – I felt suicidal.
Depression and despair can knock you out between
them.
You need to learn again how to fight against these
pressures.
I don't mean fisticuffs or physical fighting, I just mean
to stand up for yourself.
It's so easy to take a back seat and give up either to
something or to someone else.
But that's not why we're here.
We have to listen, evaluate and speak up for ourselves
and our needs.
Whilst we are convalescing from mental illness and ill
health this is often not possible.
Instead we sometimes sit and sit, unclear as to what to
do next.
I have often sat for hours, bewildered, lost in thoughts
going round and round, but really going nowhere.
It is because I had that standard provided by my carer,
to live up to, that I have gradually learned to focus
again.
I cannot always concentrate. I sometimes drift in my
mind.
Now, when I realise I'm drifting I deliberately try and
focus my mind.
I take a deep breath and say to myself that I must
concentrate.
I remember when I was first ill, the terror of losing my
mind nearly took over,

But I managed to bang the sides of the bath and make contact with myself
By loudly calling out 'you're Anne that's who you are'.
I need to remember who I have been and everything I have done.
I need to remember who I am now and how I want to live.
I need to set my goals and work on improving them gradually.
Convalescence is a gradual process.
In past times I would have been sent off to the sea for a holiday to convalesce, and get my strength back.
But that would have removed me from my living conditions
And that's not what I need when I'm convalescing.
I need to get used to my life again.

2nd June
Dear Jesus thank you for David telephoning me twice today. The first time encouraged me to be getting up and doing, and the second time just before lunch, so that he could feel OK about his break. He always seems to know when it is important to ring me and I thank him for that. Saw a couple of friends today, which is good, and they both liked my hair, after I got it cut last Friday. It's important to keep in touch with friends, and to make that effort to ring and go and see them. Mental health problems are not really well understood by people at all. It is a case of education – we need to educate others away from the stereotypical responses/reactions/attitudes.

4th June

Today at work I told my boss that I had applied for a job and put his name as referee, and it turned out he had already got the reference request. I said I didn't think the job application would come to anything, but he was encouraging and said it is good to get your hand in and to start again. He was very positive.

5th June

Today I went on a boat trip with the church prayer group. We had a lovely day out from 10 –6, with coffee and lunch, and I was given a lift home too. What more could I want. At home in the evening David asked that when we do the trip next time could he go instead, and me go to his work place.

6th June

Today I did one of the pilot project interviews, as a volunteer. Then I went shopping and tried to buy cards for my mobile phone. It still did not charge up, so maybe it is a battery it needs. I phoned both Joanie and David but neither of these changes my feelings of depression – it is with me, and it is my feelings I have to deal with. This is what I felt about before, that my feelings were not there, that I was empty. Now it is as though I have to re-learn my feelings. Dear God please help me to cope with my feelings. Thank God that David is so full of energy and also has a very good sense of humour. I thank God for the fact that he helps me and looks after me. Help me to do various things so that I can get my independence. There is a limited understanding of what it's like to be coming off anti-depressants. There is a wealth of information accumulating on Seroxat, and they include some of this on Prozac, another SSRI. Dear Jesus please help me, thank you for letting me enjoy yoga and swimming. It makes me feel more energized. I know that I need to do more of that sort of thing – it will help me. Dear God, help us all in this world to serve you, and help us lead life for all to a heavenly state. It is important to be part of a positive future. We believe in heaven and know that God wants us to arrive in heaven safely. Dear Jesus, please help us to follow your requests to follow you, and be not afraid. In this way we follow. Please lead us on.

7th June

Today we are going away for the weekend, and to collect our daughter's belongings, then to pop along to see David's parents too. Please help me to be a special person for my two children.

Wednesday 11th June

Dear Jesus, please help me to get a purpose to life so that I can be on top form. I'm glad that I can speak to some people, please help me to speak to all. Please help me.

12th June

Sometimes it is difficult for us all to cope with the demands of other people, particularly in a family where the pressures may be strong. The support of a group is also strong, and helps us to branch out. I am not forgotten just because I am less productive than the rest of the population for a while, through illness, I am not forgotten. Dear Jesus please help me to be a better mother – a stronger mother – help me to be able to stand up for what is right. Dear God help me, as you know what it is like as a parent to be strong. Imagine what a lovely surprise it was to return home and find that our son had made us a lovely meal – the 3 of us enjoyed boeuf bourgigone. If life can improve just a notch, then we will all be able to move on a pace. I think if stress becomes internalised then it leads to isolation. It was interesting today at the Platform Users Group for people with mental health experiences as a volunteer, because we had a discussion about self esteem and all the problems and difficulties. Far more useful to use the word experience which is a catchphrase and helps us to appreciate where others are coming from. Please help me to forgive the trespasses of others, and equally for them to forgive me. In the prayer group meeting today, Jesus spoke with the disciples and asked them to go out and evangelise. And he gave us the comforting words, 'For I am with you even to the end of time.' So we need to take heart and to feel that life is OK. I am really upset sometimes, but at least my mind does not wander. Watched a TV programme about a man with MND, motor neurone disease, and his demise from being cared for at home to his death, and it was a happy time in the sense that it could be, with him aware to the end, and planning for his death and care at home.

13th June
Today as usual was hard for me to get up, but at least I did. Then I did a volunteer interview for the older people project. Joanie did not get the house she was

after, so everything is on hold regarding her move. She is not coming over now to watch the tennis with me. She will be working on the prospective house this afternoon, internet searching and phoning agents. I phoned up about a job I saw advertised at the hospital and from the further information it sounds quite interesting. It is a lot of telephone work which I am quite good at, so it could be useful for me. It would also be two or three people starting at the same time, and it would not be too much pressure, as training is provided. Dear Jesus, please help me to be able to move forward in life and to survive. Help me to understand more about myself and to realise that I am a human being just like everyone else, so that I can feel similar to others, and understand what it is that makes me tick. I need to know that I am loved like other people are also loved. On the answer machine I had saved 5 messages from friends and family. I am not isolated, and I should not feel isolated. I asked David if I should send the psychiatrist an email about how I was feeling depressed, perhaps I should have more of these Natracalms, to see if they have a way of calming me down, and helping me feel less anxious and stressed. Help me be loving and kind to others – I see others all chatting away. Help me not to become withdrawn – I think that is one of my worst problems. I do not want to become withdrawn. I want an opportunity to get a job that is not too taxing, so that I can then move on from there, to develop a social life. Today I think there were 7 emails – all work and voluntary related, so I do not think that the email is necessary for me as a person. It is all work and I don't know if that is helpful for me as a person. I dread completing job application forms, because I am not in a paid job at present, and they always start off saying present job. It is depressing, as are so many other things, including my son's job, not being one which is going to take him anywhere. What will happen I wonder because there does not seem to be a plan, an overall plan.

Sunday 15th June

Today we went to yoga and swimming. After one yoga pose I was commended as having done it particularly well. That made me feel good. I enjoyed the class, it's for beginners, so it's at an easier pace than Friday's class. Please help my son to get his act together. Please let us be calm and to get things done. Help me to know how to cope with people and to speak up. Help me to speak out loud, rather than just to think. I need to be able to interact with people like my children do – help me to do this properly.
1,2,3,4,5,6,7,8,9,10,11,12,13,14,15,16,17…

On Tuesday 17th June it was our 25th wedding anniversary – the silver one. The night before we shared a bottle of champagne and also bought some flowers for a colourful bouquet for our room. On our anniversary David bought me morning tea as usual, then in the evening he got home from work early. We went for a walk in the park in the evening, then went to a Japanese restaurant for a meal, of sushi and tempura and noodles.

Thursday 19th June

Today it is a momentous occasion because our daughter left for America. This is a holiday job for some 9 weeks to be followed by travel across America. She went with her friend, who stayed here the night before their departure. She looked lovely in her little pink T-shirt with a white halter-neck underneath, and has been doing the preparatory work for it for a while now, so is absolutely ready for the trip. I will miss her and started crying, but wanted her to have a lovely time, so tried to encourage her on. She said she would ring us from New York, but I said that it would be OK just to ring on arrival. Dear God please look after my daughter who has today left for America. Please help her to be safe at all times and to enjoy and make the best of all her experiences in USA. Dear Jesus, please help me. Please help me to get to grips with my life. The sun has just come out and it's nice and sunny – a lovely day for her to fly off to America. Help her to have a lovely holiday so that she can come back with a real experience. Please help us as her parents to be able to cope with all the worries and feelings that are going on, and to support her in all these adventures.

Saturday 21st June

It is a beautiful sunny day. Heard from Joanie yesterday. She is buying a house in Kent and asked me to look up the property on the internet and tell her whether she should buy it or not. I had searched it on the net and it looked a lovely cottage with a very pretty garden, a detached house that looked idyllic in the countryside. So I said yes, and on the strength of my recommendation she put in an offer and it was accepted. So in the evening instead of going to yoga, we went over to Joanie's to celebrate with a bottle of wine and some eats. It was very pleasant and I enjoyed it. When we returned home there was a phone message to say she had arrived safely in New York and was at the camp site. Thank goodness. 5 hours behind us for the rest of the summer! Sent her an email immediately with thanks for letting us know of her safe arrival, and details of what we had been up to. I said I hoped she had a huge amount of fun, and finished with two kisses from her mum and dad. Yesterday I put in another job application – now this one is rather more high-flying – but I do not think I will get it. Our garden needs a bit of help because it is very dry and has almost become like a dust bowl in the heat. Help me to apply myself until half past one when David will be back I think.

Monday 23rd June
Today Wimbledon starts in 2 hours, so I think I'll watch it. In the old days I would have been full of excitement and enthusiasm, but these days the motivation is just not there. Why is that? Help me to accept my lot in life and to get on with it. Dear Jesus help me to be able to follow you. I need an occupation – something that will get me going, so that I can really feel that I am a worthwhile citizen. What am I supposed to do day after day. Joanie talks about having a project, and that is exactly what I need too. I need a project to get myself going. Dear Jesus please help me to find a project that would be an absorbing task. I do need to understand more about life and everything that is going on now.

David phoned me this morning about 10.30 and sounded jolly. Of course my pay packet is his pay packet, he says, these are his words to describe what I do each week. Oh dear God please help me. I'll have to get a job to take me out of myself and that that will help me to get going in the mornings. At present I feel drugged up when I wake; I suppose that is the Risperdal which is quite a strong knock-out drop. Tennis has just started. Rang Joanie just to hear her voice. She sounded happy. In the past it's always been me who has been the happy one cheering others up as I thought, but Joanie told me the other night that it was always me who was complaining. Dear God is that true? Surely not. Surely I used to phone Joanie to cheer her up and was it some kind of silly symbiosis she was talking about. I've been reading about abandonment and vulnerability and panic attacks and being dependent on a partner. What I need is a job to take me out of myself now. One aim of CBT is to help you stand back and examine ideas. When you are depressed you may tend to see everything as even worse than it really is – that is not helpful! CBT helps you come to a reasonable judgment about whether they are or are not accurate in any given situation. If you decide that you are being excessively negative, then you can look for more accurate and more helpful ways of seeing things. On the other hand if you decide that there is a real problem, then you can look for a solution to it (role of problem solving) or interpretation. Interpretation is important. If I think about it I always used to think things were better than they were – I was an optimistic sort of thinker, but in fact maybe it was just escapism. It is better to be based in reality, surely and it must be CBT which helps with this. Opinions are not facts and they can be mistaken.

Low mood

Loss of withdrawing from Pleasure/achievement activity

Vicious Circle

'I'm boring, people not talking don't like me'refusing invitations, etc.
they stop trying other people may think to approach you ,you don't like 'them'

Key Points: CBT sees depression as being closely related to certain kinds of negative thoughts and beliefs, and to their effects on your behaviour. Things that happened to you in the past may result in a tendency to think this way. By targeting these negative thoughts and changing your behaviour.
You can reduce the depression. Dear God help me to.
CBT Self-help, One step at a time.
Key points: CBT self-help approaches can help you fight back against depression. Certain features of depression can make it difficult to fight back. It is important to be prepared for these difficulties, and to approach the fight in the best way so as to give yourself the best change of succeeding. Try not to be put off by negative thoughts. Tackle recovery in small steps, one step at a time. Judge your efforts according to how you are now, not according to what you can do when you are well. Try to keep at it and slowly the enjoyment should return as well. Whatever works to lift your mood is right for you. Set small achievable targets. Give yourself a pat on the back whenever you manage

to do what you planned. Importance of physical exercise, e.g. walking, running, swimming, or other sports, can have a direct therapeutic effect on mood. It is certainly worth including in your activity planning some reasonably demanding physical exercise on a regular basis. Not only will you get fitter, but eventually you will feel better in yourself as well. Problem solving is a useful way of tackling practical problems.

I know I suffer from agitation, anxiety and general unease. Dear God please help me to cope with all this. I'm going to see the psychiatrist tomorrow for an 8 week appointment. To him I am just another appointment – one of his clients. Dear God please help him to take me seriously and to find out if there is something else he can do for me. It does say in the Prozac leaflet that you will get side effects and withdrawal effects from coming off Prozac, and one of them is anxiety. Dear God please help me to cope with this anxiety. I hate feeling anxious, this generalised feeling of anxiety. I wish just that I could cope with it all in a much better way. Joanie says to me that it is me, only me who can take control of all of this. If this is the case then I really do need to wake up and take control of all my feelings. Dear God, please help me to be able to cope. I hope my psychiatrist will care enough about me to really listen to me, and hope to be able to help me. He has had a copy of my poems, and he did share them he says with all the team. I need to be able to cope with everyday life and I seem to be failing rather miserably. I need to go and do more exercise so today I will go to Pilates Level I today.

Help me to be able to cope with this class and to get a bit of exercise.

Tuesday 24th June
Today I went to work then returned here for 1.30 to go to the psychiatrist for 2.20. David came home especially and he was here for me. He took me to the appointment where he told him that I had been suffering from depression and feeling very low. I told him that I felt it would be better if I did not have to cause all this suffering, in other words was not around, but that I had no desire to do anything about it. I told David later that I did not want to die – I want to be around. Dear Jesus help me, help me to find a niche and to have a purpose again. I need a job – not a full time one, I don't think, but one say 3 days a week. Dear Jesus help me to be strong and to be able to cope. Dear Mary, mother of Jesus, help me to be able to cope. Dear God please help me to be strong and to know whether this new anti-depressant is going to work for me. I need something to work for me so that I can cope with day to day life. Thank God that I was able to keep myself together for bringing up the children. When I saw the psychiatrist he had a student with him again, and she has been assigned to him for 5 weeks altogether. I told him that the reason he had taken me off Prozac was that it made me feel empty. He asked me whether I would rather be on/off Prozac, and I said that I didn't know, and that I was tired, after 7 years of illness. I asked him again about the lithium idea, and he said you can have lithium as well as an anti-depressant. This new anti-depressant he has prescribed for me today works on two counts, not just serotonin,

283

also is it noradrenaline, so maybe with the 2 pronged attack that will help me. I explained again to my psychiatrist that I am anxious and agitated, but that is not only off Prozac, it is on Prozac too, which does not seem to sort me out. I have been on Prozac mostly for 7 years, and I'm still depressed. Dear God, please help me to get better. I hate being anxious and having fear. Do not be afraid, for I have come to save you. Dear God please help me, please help me. In the interview my psychiatrist asked which one of us was it who didn't want the medication, as it seemed we did not want to be on medication, and I said that it was me, which it is. On the other hand, today I asked about lithium, as I said I'm tired, having been on medication and having an illness for 7 years. Dear God please help me. My mother used to call out for Jesus, Mary and Joseph, oh dear God please help me. I'm so tired after all these years and all these difficulties.

The new drug I need to take is Efexor I think. I need to see the psychiatrist again in 2 weeks so that he can see how I am before he goes off on his holiday. I need to take the first pill at breakfast time tomorrow, so that I take it at the same time each morning. I shall try and take it at 8 o'clock, because I'm a bit concerned about going in to work at 10 o'clock, and then I have a governor's meeting. I hope I do not have any adverse reaction to anything. Two friends phoned up, one about a governor's meeting and the other out of the blue which was nice. I did a picture of my left hand showing my wedding ring in my book. I phoned Joanie and told her about the new medication for me to take.

284

Another email from America, what good news, she's made some friends and is settling in.

Wednesday 25th June

Our son got up early and was doing the music in the garage again. He hopes to send his CD off to record companies. That would be good. Also he has got good knowledge now of his computer programme. I took my first new anti-depressant pill today. I hope it is good for me. It says it is a modified release capsule, so I hope that is the right thing. The pill seems to have two components, one serotonin, and the other something beginning with n. I hope it does not make me feel tired. I read the notes about it, and it says do not take alcohol, so with the orher Risperdal saying avoid alcohol, that means I will be off alcohol. Maybe that will help me lose weight too. Last night went to a Body Balance class which is a mixture of Tai Chi, Yoga and Pilates, so managed to survive it. The night before I had gone to a Pilates beginners class, and so I've now done 2 extra classes this week. I went into Crimestoppers Trust and worked from 10 until 3.30 before I went off to the governors meeting. When I came home David was here and had started making the meal for us. After dinner we went for a walk in the park, about 2 miles and I was tired when I got back. I had a little rest then I made some tea, and David did some computer work whilst I watched the tennis.

Thursday 26th June

Today I went with Joanie to see her new house. It has a lovely large cottage garden and an old barn. There are 4 bedrooms so plenty of room. There are exposed beams in the house and there is a lovely entrance hall. Joanie will need to modernise the 2 bathrooms and to completely re-do the kitchen, perhaps even opening it up by removing a wall as you come in the back door, so that the kitchen and dining room are more linked in together. She has already planned which rooms the 2 children will have. The house and garden are lovely – she will be very happy there. Also the gardener was there, so had a chat about necessary work when she owns the house. We came back and watched the tennis which was very good, then she departed for her own house. In the evening David and I went for a walk in the park again, and there was music and weight training in the garage. He has finished his demo tape but thinks he may change the vocals or get his friend to do it. I did not get along to the prayer group today, I should have phoned really, but was not sure whether I would get along after the house visit or not.

Friday 27th June

Dear God please help me not to be deceitful or hide things away from other people. I find myself lying to cover my tracks, like about what time I get up in the morning. Why? This is me deceiving myself and I feel dishonest about it all. I am afraid to say what is the truth. Dear God please help me. I have phoned up about the User Involvement Programme at our local hospital and it is an organisation service which helps you to get jobs and helps you fill in the job application form if you require it. That sounds a useful service. I phoned them and left a message for them to phone me back. It was a bit like someone said, telephone tennis, backwards and forwards, before getting anywhere. I really do want to get up and out of myself but I also need some motivation to do this. I really want to be able to do some useful paid job, not just a little computer work here and there. I wonder if there is any hope for me, and all the many others who are in these sorts of positions around the world. In the poorest countries they are concerned about their survival, so that is very different from the level of concerns we have over here. Please help me 'to be' and 'to do' dear Jesus, please help us all to do more than just survive.

Monday 30th June

Please help me to take advantage of this opportunity today at the local hospital about jobs for users of mental health services. I will be looking for work, and so they need to understand that. The fact that I have had mental health problems makes it a positive asset for me which is a very good sign. I need to be able to convince them that I could do a good job, and hope that they will be able to see this. This is an opportunity I have been waiting for a while. It is just luck sometimes when you see someone who is here, and who understands the kind of work that people who have had mental ill-health problems can do. It was a job advert I saw in the paper which told me about that job and that is a good start. I am not sure if I will be filling in lots of different job application forms today. Anyway, please help me with the task in hand. What is it I want? I need to (1) earn some money (2) do something rewarding (3) find something useful to do with my time (4) be happy (5) be respected and (6) move onwards I think. So there's a lot of different ideas there as to why I want to work and to be respected is important. I have had too much of little support now so I need to get going. I need someone to encourage me and say yes, you can do this, yes you can get into a job, yes you can be a good worker. At the weekend David and I walked round the national trust park. On the Friday evening we went to the social club party and took our friend along. Please let me find a job where I will be helpful to some of the people there. It is a good idea to have people who have experience of mental health problems because they are sympathetic to the needs of people who have been there at some point in their lives too. I need to move on and get into some sort of useful job now. Please help me. David has been talking about looking for a new job, and perhaps the two of us need to get ourselves more organised now in that way. It becomes difficult for us to be able to get work though, because of our age, although we have more skills and experience now.

Friday 4th July

I'm starting to feel a bit better now on this Efexor, so there must be some benefit in medication sometimes. This week there have been two results of my job applications. One said I was unsuccessful and thanked me for my application and would keep my CV on file, and the other said I was invited along for an interview. I'll have to show that I can be a good team player, as that was the criticism last time. Also I need to brush up a bit on my computer programmes. I don't know how but I can try. More news from America, although she has been in the infirmary with a fever, but is OK now. Dear God thank you for looking after our daughter and helping her to have a good time on holiday and at work.

I wish that our son cold settle into getting a good job and use his skills and do well. My job referee phoned to say that she had got the request for a reference for me. If only I can get the job. I need to be able to get myself up in the mornings, and get ready for work. I will need to enlist the help of David to get me up, so that I feel motivated to get myself ready. At work need to eat fruit and try and lose weight, because I am desperately trying to control my consumption of foods, so that I become fitter and lose some weight. Sent an email to America and got my CV together. Phoned the two local employment agencies who take on secretaries as temporaries and they advised to send in my CV. Dear Jesus please help me to be able to cope with all these things – there is so much to do and I need to make a start on it. I'm beginning to feel a bit better I think on Efexor, and beginning to think that I could work again, which is what I need to do. Maybe I have had more of a generalized anxiety disorder, and because I did not press that enough with the psychiatrist, then I ended up not getting that dealt with as an important thing for me. I need to be able to value myself in society amongst everything that is going on, as well as in the home. To me, the central force of my life is my home life and that has ruled everything I have done. I probably needed to be on the anxiety pill before, it's just that I didn't know that I was more anxious than most people so I was not aware that I had to do something about it. Dear God please help me to be able to cope with all of this because it is now building up. When I first started at Crimestoppers Trust, it was all I could do to get through the day, but now it is just a small part of my week. The balance seems to have changed, and I'm beginning to feel much more positive. Yes, I think the world does need me, so I am pleased to be here and to be able to cope with my life in a way that was so much better than before. In a way it is just the beginning of everything again. Dear Jesus, please let me be strong and be able to cope with everything that is going on.

Tuesday 8th July
I had my appointment today with the psychiatrist and he said to carry on Efexor as it seemed to suit me. I take the same dose of 2 x 75g tablets. He also suggested I might like to join the lifestyle and diet class at 3.30 pm on a Monday for an hour. He said he will make a referral for me, and I said I would go providing I did not get a job in the meantime. I asked about work and he said that would be good for me. I said I didn't really have any motivation, and that perhaps having a job would help that. I explained that I had been very involved in looking after my children, and that now they are grown up and there's a gap needing to be filled which would probably be helped if I could get a job. I told him I had an interview at the local hospital next week and he asked me about my typing speeds, which I said are very good. He does not need to see me again until 18th August. So I think it was a successful appointment again, as a follow-on from last time. The medical student was in the room again. He asked me about the exercise I have each week, and I told him about the yoga and swimming, but he does not think seriously that yoga is exercise, as it is all keeping still, so I explained that it was stretching and breathing. He also explained about eating low fat and low sugar diet and said these topics were covered on the diet and

lifestyle group. Of course I know about eating well, but knowing and doing are two separate things. He asked me if I thought I had put on weight on Efexor, but I do not think so, in fact I have a slightly flatter stomach as I have already been eating fruit. Another good thing the Dr suggested was to take a walk of about 20 minutes to half an hour. Also that you can eat tomatoes and carrots as much as you like, and also eat fruit. The trouble with these anti-depressants is that they increase the appetite, so the class is run especially for people who are on medication like me. I've tried to keep active today, as that is another important factor. Dear God please help me to do more so that I do not get fat.

Friday 11th July
I've been feeling really de-motivated and don't know what I can do to help myself. It has been so hot, too hot to go out at all, or do anything, or end up in a pool of sweat. I have drunk lots of water. Dear Jesus please help me. I need to trust in you and have hope, so please help me to do so. David is home now, so I feel better, thank God. Please help me to manage the yoga class as I often get tired in that.

Monday 14th July
I am determined to lose weight. I hate being so tired in the hot weather and being too heavy to do things. I managed quite well at yoga. It was an inspiration to me that I did all the sun salutations. It could be because I did one round of them at home before I left, it could be because I prayed, or it could be because I was more determined. It could be because of the sunshine or because the teacher introduced it saying we would do it

slowly. Sometimes on the Sunday class we have a chance to do the salutations at our own speed which is an inspiration to me too. This morning I drank a lot of water and I think the best thing to do is drink water, because it will clear me out and it will be good for my health, and it will take the edge off my appetite, and a useful way of filling my stomach. They do say that it is important to drink, rather than eat. Again I will also make sure that I do not have much alcohol. I have learned that I can cope with my feelings without alcohol, I do not need to drown myself in my feelings, by drowning my body in alcohol. Dear God please help me to really cut down on everything I eat. It is so much easier in the summer to manage that. It is easier to just not eat. The only worry is that if I do not eat, my body will start to store what it does eat for fat supplies.

Had a nice time at the weekend, and we spent time at the river and the parks nearby. On the Saturday after a walk we went to the open air swimming pool, and managed to have two little swims in the slow lanes and dried off in between in the sunshine. It was very pleasant and absolutely packed out. It was obvious that everyone enjoys the open air pool on such a beautifully hot day. Then we ate out by the Thames in a riverside pub. We drank a Pimms which was nice then ordered a meal, and thoroughly enjoyed the evening out – it was very good for us. Then on Sunday we went along to the Hampton Court Flower Show – very expensive and difficult to find areas in the shade in the extreme heat. Some of the laid out gardens were lovely and well worth seeing. The show was completely packed out and there were loads of coach parties there too. Dear Jesus please help me to lose weight, <u>please, please, please</u>. It is so easy for some of these really thin people to be able to do exercise – it has never been easy for me, so I need to lose weight, and feel better. I will stop taking tea, with milk so much, and other caffeine drinks, and try and drink more water.

25th July

It is one week since David's father died. He died last Friday afternoon in the Royal Free Hospital in Camden area. He had come down to London en route to France for a party weekend, a 21st birthday party. Three of them were going off together, when he took ill, luckily in a doctor's surgery, as he went to pick up a prescription for his diabetic medicines. He had a heart arrest and was revived by the doctors before he was taken to the hospital. His daughter had been with him in the surgery when he collapsed and after remaining with him whilst the doctors set to work, she returned home to collect her mother, his wife of 61 years, to bring her to see him. He managed to squeeze her hand on her arrival, then was taken to the hospital. Again he had to be revived en route and they thought he was dead, but he started breathing again. Then he was put on a life support machine and given drugs to help his recovery. David, his sister Fiona and his mother were there all day with him, and in the evening, David and I went up together to see him and to be with his mother. We saw his dad unconscious but breathing through the life support system with the help of a respirator. He seemed to me to be relaxedly breathing, but it was the effect of the drugs and the machinery. He had had a bad turn in the afternoon, and was now totally dependent on the machine for breathing. We stayed there until 11.30 pm then went home. In the morning David went to work, but Fiona telephoned with the bad news that the doctors were saying that with their agreement they were stopping the drugs, and it was a question of turning off the life support system, and that he was not expected to survive. So, we set off again for the hospital , a journey of an hour or more and arrived to find a completely different scene. The family were assembling from different parts of the country, the other side of London, Birmingham, Kent, Swansea and Liverpool. Later, after everyone who could be there had assembled to say their goodbyes, the life support system was turned off and David's dad died when they took him off. Everyone was there who could be there. In the circumstances of his being travelling en route to France he had a good send off. He had no pain, and his death was quick. Altogether there were 5 of his 8 children at his bedside as he died, as well as his wife. There were also 3 partners there, a husband, a wife (me) and a long-term friend. David's mother was very comforted by the fact that so many of his children were at his bedside. Before 3.00 pm the Doctor and Nurse came to talk to the family and said they were switching off the life support system with agreement of the family but they could not say how long he would live. In fact he died pretty quickly, almost immediately. Everyone saw him died, then the doctors removed all the tubes and the pipes and we could see him without the machinery, dead. Even his grand-daughter was there at that point to say good-bye to her grandfather. We had spent most of the last 36 hours in the relatives room at the hospital, so these facilities are important for families. David said a prayer for his father round the bedside as did Fiona. We all joined in, as best we could. It was a lovely way to say goodbye in these circumstances. Then, after collecting his belongings we all made our way to Fiona's house and had tea. Everyone made their way back to the family home from there, and there was a family reunion in Banbury on the Saturday. Both the two remaining living sons and their families turned up there too, so everyone was there. It was very moving, and it was what David's mother had wanted. She had found the family photos which were mainly taken by David's dad, and we spent many hours admiring them. A family member offered to put them all on to a CD so that everyone could have a copy. In the evening we all sat down to a lovely chicken meal which David's brother, the chef had prepared. We toasted David's dad with 2 bottles of champagne for the assembled group. We knew we would all meet again at the funeral when that was arranged.

Now that was the last entry in my journal. I think it is interesting that I decided to stop writing a journal entry on the death of David's father, considering my journal entries and my book have largely been about the death of my mother. It is quite a symmetrical end to my journaling. But of course, although David knew that I had lost a parent too, it is so different to lose a parent when you are an established adult, and the person who died is aged 83. That does not devalue the death or the life of the person who has passed away, rather it says that we need to remember our parents for what they did, and how they were a part of our lives. It is obviously so much easier if you have a parent who has lived to the well established age of 83 as opposed to the age of 56, like my mother. Straight away we were able to laugh and joke about David's father and tell stories of his life and his achievements. He had been a wine connoisseur so it was totally appropriate that we toasted him the day after his death in champagne, the champagne he had bought for the family anyway. He was very generous and family minded. I found that very strange, to be toasting in champagne after a death, when my mother's death had produced a Scottish wake, and then withdrawal into our own lives, and in a sense a running away from what had really happened. David's father's death also really made us all aware how alone now his wife of over 60 years was – now she was a widow and expected to carry on her life without her constant companion of these many years. I was amazed at how she talked about her husband and was the one to lead the toast to him, and through that I learned a valuable lesson. She had lived her life to the full with him and was now able to carry on without him because of that strength. She passed that on to us too. The routine continued. The meals, the washing, the cleaning, the church attendance, everything so far as was humanly possible. I asked one of David's sisters how his mother could carry on like that, simply sticking to the tasks that had to be done, and she said to me that it was important to keep to the routine. I had never thought of it like that before, and I found it all so totally different from the way that my family had reacted, by running away really to a new life. To some extent it was circumstances and the age of the bereaved which made the difference. At 21 and 18 we are just beginning life and looking forward to what we can achieve, and in our 80's we are pleased to celebrate life's achievements and those of our long-standing partners. David's father's death has been a positive experience for me. There have been many stories about his father which we may not have heard before, and everyone is talking about the long and good life he lead. I think it is sad and so does David, that his dad could not have rallied and lived a little bit longer as companion to his mother, who seems so full of life and energy. But that was his time, as it was for my mother all those years ago, when she had merely achieved the age of 56 years. This is life. And that is what I have learned. We all need to go forward with the help of our friends and companions and meet life as it evolves. We are all part of that life and living, and not passive participants or active rebellers. To me it is so important that we live life to the full when we are alive and share it with those we know. Perhaps that is what will give me my motivation for life in the future. I need to move on and will again learn from David and all the other people I meet how to.

As a postscript may I add how David has been so attentive to his mother since his father's death. He has additionally phoned his mother several times a week, to keep in touch and make sure she was OK. She is lucky with a large family of children because she has had contact with most of her family throughout this time, everyone doing what they could. David has taught me how important it is to keep in contact with the family and I have learned a lesson from this. I have been trying to phone my father on a more regular basis, to ensure that he is OK and just to hear his news and relay mine. After all he is now in his late 80's and is managing superbly on his own since the death of his second wife now some 8 or so years ago. It is amazing how the human being learns to adapt. Of course we all learn as we go along. However, I have still not learned how to communicate effectively with my second sister, who lives her life quite separately in Scotland's capital city without regular calls, letters or news passing to her sisters. There's nowt so queer as folk the saying goes, and certainly we live and learn so far as family goes.

Chapter 26 - Time To Catch Up

The other stage of moving on for me has been the end of my time as a full-time and active mother. My two children are now quite independent and starting to live their own lives. I want them to be happy and seek out their challenges in life just as I have done. A university education has been a good starting point, and then their attempts to gain work experience, travel and create their own friendships have been other roads for them to start travelling. For me this has had a profound effect upon my way of living. I was always very involved as a mother, perhaps too involved in a way, because I did tend to centre my life around that of my two children, and their schooling, and their existence. Our holidays were exciting adventure type holidays to broaden their minds, and their school work and the school term was very important in my eyes. To a large extent our social life revolved round the school activities and their friendships, along with our extended family. We were always busy, and on top of this came my work. After the children were born I did go back to outside paid work but I found it a great strain to carry on the kind of advice work and practical support which I had been doing prior to having my family. So I left my job and some years later set up my own business working from home doing secretarial services. This worked fine for some 6 years, looking after the children and family and working in my business too. I brought in money, maintained my confidence and self-esteem and had an outside interest. I stopped the business when we moved house about 2 years before I had my breakdown, and a year later I also handed in my notice in the little part time management job I had taken on. Once more I was working at home, but this time helping my husband in his business which was now run from home, and at the same time looking after the children and family commitments. Then in 1997 I had my breakdown and became a case for the psychiatric community team. David my husband took over a large part of the care for the children whilst I was really ill, and so my emphasis shifted with me trying to take care of myself. I was not very clever at that then, and felt very guilty about not being able to look after the children as I would have liked. But over the years I have adapted to this re-balancing of my life and the children no longer being the centre of my existence. The 'empty nest syndrome' has been very difficult for me. It has taken time, but is good for all of us. No longer am I trying to be this supermum and to be all things to all people, but I give my children, now young adults the space they need to get on with their own lives. It has been hard to make these adjustments to my life, but I think the process is almost complete.

Chapter 27 - The Use of Alcohol as Self-Medication

When I started reading the story of Patty Duke and her manic depression, early on in her story she talked about alcohol and the use of it as an attempt at self-medication. I had never come across that concept before but I do think it has applied to me at times. Over the years I think I have attempted to use alcohol to de-stress from the pressures of work and home life, as you often read people do. In the last seven or so years, I have had times where I have been off alcohol altogether, as a deliberate attempt to lose weight, drinking basically only water and tea. Then I have a break from that routine and enjoy some wine again, and sometimes get into the habit of drinking more wine than the recommended units of alcohol for women. So, then I take another break and go on to tea and water again, and do not find it too much of a problem. The only thing is I do enjoy wine to drink as I enjoy a fine meal, and again both of these add on the weight. So, as part of my nutrition I do try and reduce consumption of comfort eating foods, high fat foods and wine.

The last time I saw a psychiatrist he said it seems 'she has a problem' in the sense that I was drinking half a bottle of wine at least 5 nights a week. This is not good news, but it is probably true. I have sort of become rather dependent upon a drink of wine in the evenings. Is it in the same sort of way that I am dependent upon my husband for support and help, or is it just a habit and easily available? It is so easy to slip into patterns of behaviour, addictive or otherwise, and we need to be vigilant about what we are thinking and doing. I will make a conscious effort to watch what I drink more carefully and try to sharpen up on my behaviour. The psychiatrist suggested noting a drinks diary, to keep an exact note of what alcohol I am drinking. To be very clear though, I do not drink spirits at all – only wine. There is quite a bit of medical opinion around which says that a glass or two of a red wine is a healthy addition to our diets. It is like my mother always said, 'Moderation in all things.' But it is often noted that Bipolar II people – like me – often have a problem with alcohol. Is this a problem we need to address.

Chapter 28 – The Power of Prayer

I have referred in my narrative to the prayer group which I attend on a regular weekly basis and have done for the last year. Praying does provide an answer to worries and cares, by helping you to refocus and think more positively on the problems presented to you in life. There is the social aspect to prayer at regular weekly Masses which I also attend, and the friendships which you establish as a result of going to the prayer group and social club activities. Prayer does have an important role to play for me in my life and being invited along to the prayer group meeting did open my eyes to the power of prayer. Over the last year I have learned a great deal about my need for quiet time, and prayer, and this has helped me use my time more efficiently. From this, I can now view life more positively, so although my life is ostensibly the same, the power of prayer has changed it round for me.

Chapter 29 - Therapy and A Productive Life

I do now feel that my self-help therapy through writing has been a very positive step for me. Nobody suggested that I should write a book, it was just my own need to get my ideas down which prompted the project. Also searching on the internet I have found that there are other books available from people who have felt the need to write about their mental health experiences. Put in a search on the topic you may be interested in and then you will find a selection of books to choose from. It is also quite useful to look at the websites of the various mental health groups that exist, and something else I have found recently is a mental health conference on the web, which invites you to read various mental health papers and then join in the debate on mental health services and the user/survivor issues.

I have read quite a number of books about mental health but the best I have found is 'Going Mad? Understanding Mental Illness' by Michael Corry and Aine Tubridy. It has excellent descriptive pieces about the various kinds of mental health problems that there are. I read this when I was quite manic and I felt as though I had everything in the book to a greater or lesser extent. But I found it very reassuring that the symptoms I was experiencing were known well enough to be written about. It is useful to read about other people's experiences and this is where I hope that my book will help here too.

I see this book, my story as a step forward for me. Along with making the effort to get into part-time work again, through registering with an employment agency, I feel I am starting to take a stand with my life. After seven years of ups and downs with depression and mania, and mental illness, this is really good news. I have maintained faith in the medical profession who have referred me when necessary to the specialist psychiatric services and continued with prescribed medication, while encouraging me to take on the challenge of work. When I spoke once with my psychiatrist and said sometimes I got really worried about even going for a walk, he said to me the thing to do was just to get on with it and do the walk. Sometimes that is easier said than done, but I have found that on this anxiety reducing drug I am more able to take such decisions. I feel more positive, and success breeds success, so I feel it is a rolling process of improvement. I have been through quite a lot one way or another, and so have a lot of experience which has helped me to grow too. I have used my own version of behaviour therapy in searching for answers to help me change my behaviour – my readings and writings have been very productive here.

I am one of the lucky ones who has always had my family there to encourage and support me. They have been interested in my journaling and are now interested in my book. But most of all they are interested in me, and how I am doing. Both my son and my daughter want to see me getting on with life, and achieving things in a productive life. How often has my husband said to me that my input has been essential, when I have described myself as being useless. These thoughts have been my mainstay when I felt down. Now I need to strive to make sure that I carry on with this more fulfilling life.

Chapter 30 – Remembering My Mother – Some Positive Images

One of the photographs of my mother I have chosen for this book is one that was taken in her service years, some time before she married and gave birth to me. She would probably be in her late 20's at the time, because I think she was 33 years old when she had me. Her photograph looks lovely, she looks full of life and her eyes show that interest in everything around her. She always had an opinion on what was going on and was well read. She looks so smart and so slim in her uniform. Another photograph I would like to include is that of my parents on their wedding day – they looked good together – 1st April 1950. Now I remember my mother took me to school everyday until I was old enough to go alone, at about the age of 9, because in those days it was safer to travel on the roads, there were less cars. She accompanied me on my first day and gave me the courage to go in and face the rest of the class and the whole school. I did not know anyone else, but I do not remember crying at all. Maybe leaving children at school was a lot more brutal in those days. I also remember my mum being there at home all the time for me and my sisters. She did not go out to work but was always there in the home, as was quite usual in the 1950's. So, although she had had a good university training and a responsible job before she married, she became a housewife and looked after her three children at home. She organised the household and everything centred around her – she was the life force. I remember if she was a bit cross about anything, then the whole household had to tread warily until we were back on an even keel again.

Life at home was happy. Here is a photograph of my mother's three children – all together in a row. We led a quiet life, of going to school then returning home for tea, which was always laid out on the table for us. Then we all had a family supper when my dad came home from work. Our maternal grandfather was there all the time too until his death when I was 12. We sometimes went to the cinema with our mother, and there were the occasional outings to the theatre, but otherwise we had a quiet life at home. My parents did not do much entertaining, so there were not frequent visitors to the home. But my mum wanted the three girls to grow up independently, so she would encourage us to go off to the library to change our library books, or to go off on a cycle ride, or to play with our friends across the road. Sometimes our friends came round to play too. I remember my mother cooking – sometimes she would have a whole ox tongue boiling in a pan of water, the smell was awful and I hate ox tongue to this day. At Christmas she used to receive a large chicken or turkey by post and it was necessary to take all its feathers out, and then prepare it for the oven. We used to help my mum prepare the Christmas cake and just loved to taste the cake mix. On a Saturday evening we all had a supper trolley meal watching a good film or series on the TV – that was fun. Every Sunday for lunch we would have a proper cooked meal, and quite often it would be my turn to make the custard trifle for the desert, and whip up the cream, which I enjoyed. When I went to senior school, my mum would help me with my homework, especially when I first started mathematics which I found hard. In time I became confident enough to do my own work without assistance, but I always knew she was there if I needed any help. On Sundays we would go to church with my mum to the little local church of St Christopher's.

I was 14 when my mum developed heart trouble and soon after we moved to Scotland. We, the children lived with our grandmother and great aunt, and my parents stayed for 3 months in a hotel near my dad's work HQ. Then we all crowded together into the house for the rest of the year, before my parents bought a family house for us. That was special when we got our own house again, and we had our parents to ourselves. My mum settled us all in and we set about family life again. We had a couple of years before the heart trouble struck again, and this time was quite fun. I was a teenager and liked to go out and about with my friends, but I was well behaved and did not cause my parents any grief. Not so my middle sister, who did tend to be rather more difficult. But we all got on. I was particularly close to my youngest sister, and we are regularly in touch to this day. For a further two years my mum's ill health affected the family in a large way, but we learned to just cope. At 18 I went off to university and my two sisters were left at home with my mum who was by that time really suffering from her heart trouble. Three years later she had died, but we all learned to get on with our lives. She had taught us to be independent thinkers and survivors in the world.

When I started this book I thought it was going to be just about me and my manic depression, but it turned into a much wider story, as no doubt it should. For the first time, with my journaling I began to express my feelings about my mother, and her early death in my life. Simultaneously I began to explore my grief, through readings which I unconsciously sought out. I mean I did not go out to find a book on bereavement, but somehow my searches took me to those books, which dealt with loss and grief surrounding death, as well as all the other emotions which arise around important events in life. With the framework in place I was enabled to write about how I had felt at the time of my mother's death, and my subsequent loss of my baby at miscarriage. I realised I had buried these feelings and run away from them, just trying to get on with life. But it had to come out in the end in my writings. Then, I gradually moved into the whole area of self-esteem and self development which also featured heavily in my journaling. I referred particularly to my psychiatric treatment and the various alternative therapies like complementary therapy and counselling which I took up. It has been a road I have travelled with the help of my family and friends and the various groups and organisations I have been involved with along the way. I could not have done this alone.

Chapter 31 – Death in the Family

My own father David Blaikie, died on 14th December 2003. His death was totally unexpected and very sudden. He was talking to us and alive and well one day and then overnight he died. We had no preparation for his death at all, and so it came as a sudden jolt to all our senses. Death in this way seems a peaceful event for the person who has passed away, but leaves others saddened and at a loss to understand what has happened. My father was the kindest and gentlest of men, and had lived a long and fulfilled life, in the business community until retired from work, then serving the community, with his charity work in the local area, including the church and the youth club, and most especially his work with the national Scottish Boys Clubs. But particularly, my father was important in our family life as a grandfather to his six grandchildren, four boys and two girls, who all loved him dearly. For me, and for my two sisters, this has been another step in the process of assuming responsibility for our lives – we are now the older generation – we are the ones to whom others look for answers and for companionship. My father's death has also left us as orphaned adults, which is a great theme for many writers trying to understand the demise of their parents. For me, I have been living a life independent from my father for a long time, with my husband and two children, so I do not feel like an abandoned orphan as some adults do at this time. Rather I felt these feelings years and years ago, when my mother died. For me, it is a time of quiet contemplation and thoughts of peace. For me the circle is complete. My mother died, my father remarried, my step-mother died and then my father has now died. Their circle is now at peace. So I too can be at peace.

For many years I had the feeling of death in the family, and it was very difficult for me to be able to see the fruits of life. The house where my mother lived and died has always been a sad place for me, even though it resounded with the sounds of happy grandchildren again with the arrival of my step-mother and the new generation. However, the house passed again into sadness after the death of my step-mother, and finally has sounded the death knoll with my father's passing. It is time for the house to move on to another young family, where the sound of laughter will once again be heard within its walls. For me, I have my happy memories of life in the house with all the holidays with the grandchildren staying with their grandparents, and the happiness they brought each other.

For my two children in particular it has been one of the saddest of years for them. They have lost two grandfathers, both in their 80's. For children it is a time of change when a grandparent dies. In one case, that of my father, his house will be sold and all the contents be distributed or sold. It is truly the end of an era in that place at that time. The onus is now on myself and my husband to look after the children and the family. No more can we depend upon the guidance and love which has passed down to us from the other older generation. For my husband's family, the extended family circle continues. The children have one surviving grandparent, their paternal grandmother, who is still continuing her life as before in the family home, caring at a distance for all the sons, daughters, and the grandchildren who are starting to find their way in life. But she is now equally dependent upon her own children for interaction and day to day comfort. This goes to show how we all are interdependent each upon the other in our lives and we need the contact with others to grow. We need to move forward, for ourselves but especially for our own children, the grandchildren, for yet a little longer. We need to reinforce our kinship ties and remember our inheritance. 'No man is an island.' We all need each other.

For me, I am now part of the older generation. I no longer have a parent, except my husband's mother. I have grown into being the older generation for my children and their friends. I need to learn to live up to this position and be able to provide at least a part of that solace which they need to sustain themselves. I need to help provide the solidarity and continuity which is so essential.

Having Manic Depression by Anne Brocklesby

I hate being ill dammit.
I hate it.
Yes, why am I like this?
It's so bloody frustrating.
Sometimes I can just speak up for myself and say
what I want to say.
Other times I feel like a mouse, scared, timid alone
in a big world.
Now I don't tell everyone about it.
In fact, very few people know.
I'm scared to talk about it in a general sense,
because of the kind of rejection I fear.
I must say even family members do not understand.
They seem to have lost contact with me.
I mean I am still here, but only my own immediate
family seem to understand.
My two children, and above all, my husband, my
carer, my crutch.
With others – can I make the effort?
If yes, it's OK.
Otherwise I'm cut off.
It seems to depend so much on me.
For a while I tried desperately to keep in touch with
'family' members and wrote
letters and cards.
I can honestly say that basically they were ignored.
No one replied.
So now I've stopped.

Except for those members who equally feel the need to communicate, who also I see have mental health difficulties too.
I have learned a lesson.
Fine when I'm well and can deal with them equally.
But otherwise no.
We have two very different families.
So really I am quite isolated.
My husband bears the brunt of my condition and does his best to keep me going.
We have few friends.
I have met a few people, mostly with mental health problems who I talk to.
Everything else is superficial.

Is this the stigma that everyone talks about?
We feel it.
Stigma becomes a part of us, and so that is what we expect.
It becomes our own little world.
There are few friends.
There is no real work – only voluntary work.
My friendship circle is severely restricted and I mean severely.
Here life is quiet.
So there is a lot of isolation and I suppose that is stigma.
It is a form of perception, as is eyesight problems, which I also have.
So inside and out there is stigma.
Help do not desert me.
Reach out to me too please.
Now I am one of the stigmatised.

Help me – help me!!

NB   Could also call this poem 'Stigma'

Exercise Is Not That Easy by Anne Brocklesby

No, exercise is not that easy.
Not if it takes you a while to get out of bed in the
morning that is.
You need to find the motivation from somewhere to
get up and go for it.
Where is that necessary force – deep within.
How can we find it?
Try a little exercise and see.
Just one or two minutes is a good starting point.
A bit of a walk is another.
Every day do something.
Try to do a little more each day, and build it up to a
respectable amount.
Even if at first all you can do is walk to the shops
and back, that is something.
It is a good thing to be able to do.
There are many people who are housebound, or who
feel that they cannot go out.
Agoraphobia is a terrible condition to have, where
you are too afraid to leave the house.
You spend all your time at home, because it is safe,
and feel in a panic if you should go out, or even the
thought of going out.
Fear and panic need to be controlled too.

Sometimes medication is the answer, we can pop another pill which provides a bit of tranquillity, or take some of those soothing teas.

Perhaps they will provide an answer to the condition, and enable us to be positive, and to venture forth.

A quick solution may be all that we have time for in the sense of achievement.

We need to do.

So, if we need to go out and we want to go out, we will try one of those medicated solutions.

But, if we have lost the motivation to go out for a visit to the shops, or to meet up with a friend, then it is all too difficult.

At that stage it might be too much to plan a visit out at a regular time, and so we gradually become more housebound, as we fear, and are afraid to go out.

Fear not said the angel. Do not be afraid said Jesus to his disciples.

Fear is one of the modern curses of all time.

So instead of being on the treadmill of fear, and trepidation, we need to move to get out to the gym to be on the treadmill there, or to go for a walk in our local neighbourhood.

It just takes us to start somewhere, to see a bit of an improvement.

We need to be able to build on the position where we are, in other words to take a few more steps.

It's a bit like a child who learns how to build bricks, because we need to learn how to make those moves to improve our fitness.

Exercise is not that easy when you have been ill with mental illness, and one of the major problems is motivation to do anything.

Then, exercise becomes more important, because we are likely just to have been sitting still anyway, sitting thinking or doing nothing.

It is important to be able to think and to do.

We cannot spend all our lives being introspective, thinking about what we should do, but never motivating ourselves to do it.

Exercise is not that easy if you have mental health problems, because the motivation to exercise is just not there.

But, start somewhere, maybe even devising a little fitness programme of your own, that you could do in the house, just to get yourself going in the morning.

Or make that special effort to get out to the gym for a class which you know that you will be able to do, a class for your level.

There are aqua classes which help you to exercise in water, where the water takes the main weight, especially if you are feeling very heavy and unmotivated.

The feel of the water can be soothing.

The lift from the volume of the water can be uplifting.

The gentle feel of pushing your way through water may be just what you need to get those senses going again.

When we have mental health problems we usually notice that our senses go down, and perhaps we need to stimulate one sense to liven up the rest.

The sense of touch could be used, by using the water, to gently lift and protect the movements of the tired body.
Then perhaps a yoga class, where there are gentle movements and breathing
Exercises which again can be used to stimulate the senses and relax the mind.
A body balance class could help us move that bit more to learn again how to feel the body moving in different directions and the power of the limbs to carry us forward.
Or a class in meditation, with breathing and movement.
Exercise is not that easy when you have mental health problems, but we do need to try and start somewhere.
A walk each day, a bit of an exercise class, a swim, some yoga.
Try it and see.

Just Convalescing by Anne Brocklesby

David says I'm convalescing – I don't know.
I've been unwell for so long, it becomes a way of life.
That's why it's so important to have a standard to live up to.
And I mean to grow towards it.
I intend to make progress towards my goal of independence,
At present and over the last few months I have had so many ups and downs – it's like a roller-coaster.
One minute I'm OK, the next I'll be dissolving in tears in temporary despair,

Of course now it could be cold turkey – coming off
Prozac, which I've been on for 7 years almost
continuously, and now off it for the last 4 weeks.
It's not so severe as last summer, when I was on
Prozac and came off Risperdal – I felt suicidal.
Depression and despair can knock you out between
them.
You need to learn again how to fight against these
pressures.
I don't mean fisticuffs or physical fighting, I just
mean to stand up for yourself.
It's so easy to take a back seat and give up either to
something or someone else,
But that's not why we are here.
We have to listen, evaluate and then speak up for
ourselves and our needs.
Whilst we are convalescing from mental illness and
ill health this is often not possible.
Instead we sometimes sit and sit, unclear as to what
to do next.
I have often sat for hours, bewildered, lost in
thoughts going round and round, but really going
nowhere.
It is because I had that standard provided by my
carer to live up to, that I have gradually learned to
focus again.
I cannot always concentrate.
I sometimes drift in my mind.
Now, when I realise I'm drifting I deliberately try
and focus my mind.
I take a deep breath and say to myself I must
concentrate.

I remember when I was first ill, the terror of losing my mind nearly took over, but I managed to bang the sides of the bath, and make contact with myself by loudly calling out, "you're Anne that's who you are".

And I put my hands to my face to feel it, and to gently pat the skin.

I need to remember who I am now and how I want to live.

I need to set my goals and work on improving them gradually.

Convalescence is a gradual process.

In past times I would have been sent off to the sea for a holiday to convalesce and get my strength back.

But that would have removed me from my living conditions.

And that's not what I need when I'm convalescing.

I need to get used to my life again.

Fear Of Living by Anne Brocklesby

Today I received details of my life insurance endowment policy – they will pay over £26,000 if I should die.

Big deal – that is not all I'd be to my family should I die.

Heaven forbid that I should died, but why am I so scared of living.

I have this fear of life, sometimes I am so scared, I just do not want to do things,

I fear the consequences of my actions, and what other people think about me or what I should do.

Why is this?

I have always been anxious, even as a child, and I do not know what else to say about it.

Why should I have been so anxious?

Well I was the oldest daughter of 3, and my mother was a very strong minded woman.

However, she became ill soon after the death of her father, she developed heart trouble, and for a time she went into hospital so we lived at home on our own.

Not entirely alone, but our father would come home from work, after he had visited her in hospital so it would be late.

I had been used to a family life with my grandfather there too, so it was very quiet.

Suddenly I was the oldest, and I mean the oldest person around, at 13 for quite a bit of the time, and it was a bit scary.

I mean I had to take responsibility for my sisters, even though they did not want me, their older sister to tell them what to do.

Yet one of my sisters, the youngest tells me she looked up to me, so what I did was important.

The only trouble is that I think it is this caring role, as a young carer for my sisters, and also for my father, and then on her return my mother, which has caused this anxiety.

I would always worry about everyone.

I saw that as my job.

Yet, at 13, 14, 15 and 16 I should have been rebelling, having fun as a teenager, and doing all those things which other youngsters did.

On the whole this was not the case for me, we were alone, and pretty lonely.

I did not have many friends.

When we moved up to Scotland, when I was 14, I formed two close friendships and they guided me through my teenage years.

Before that I had been pretty alone in my London school, a large grammar school.

I did not talk about my family with my acquaintances, so I was left to deal with it alone. And for me that was alone.

Then again as an older teenager, my mother was ill again, and we had to learn to live with the fact that she had heart disease.

Life was always fraught for me, and I used to be a very well behaved daughter so as not to cause any problems for my parents.

Fat lot of good that did me in my caring role as a developing teenager, and is something which has affected me to this day.

When I was 21, after my mother's death, I wanted to have some fun.

I chose a serious job, being a social worker, but in my private life I did have some fun.

This was the important part of starting out on life for me, and soon I met my husband and we became friends on the path of life together.

After my own children became teenagers, I too became ill, and had a nervous breakdown, which does not seem surprising if you know about my propensity to worry.

I worried about my children and that they would grow up safe and well.

I found it hard being a mother, something I could never relax into.

Day by day I managed fine, because I was organised and could keep control.

After I had my nervous breakdown the children were supervised as teenagers, more by their father, which let me have a break from the caring role.

This has done me the world of good, and I have gradually learned to stand back.

Change worries me, and I am trying to work out why.

It must be the memories and the associations I have with my past, that when there was change, it was usually for the worse.

So, now I need to re-programme my brain, and think positively.

I go to a Prayer Group once a week on a Thursday with Father Mitchell, and there we learn about the power of prayer, and learn not to be afraid.

This has been very supportive to me over the last year, when I have felt extremely vulnerable.

There have been so many times over the last few years that I have been truly afraid of living, and consequently afraid of dying.

I became so worried that things were going to happen to my family, that I could not let them out of my sight.

I used to worry my daughter would get into difficulties when she was out.

I used to worry that my son would not be able to get himself through university and into a job.

Through prayer I have learned to accept and renew my faith.

I have learned to take each new day.
I still need to learn to love life again and to be positive.
I always thought before that I was positive and always looking on the bright side, but rather I think I was fearful.
We need to learn that it is the little things which make up life, and we need to learn to like the little things.
For me it is a bit like learning everything again.
This time, it is slowing down, and learning to appreciate the little everyday things.
Before I would always be planning ahead for what was to come, so that I maintained total control of the situation.
Now, I have learned to sit back and to some extent take what comes.
What I need in the end of course is a balance, which is enjoyment of the day to day routine, and planning ahead for routine and also enjoyment.
Help me to be able to focus on enjoying life and living it well.

Finding A New Way Ahead by Anne Brocklesby

I remember the day when I nearly lost my head, when I wondered if I was Anne any more.
I had to pat my face, and call out my name to myself, to wake myself up or whatever else it took just to get in touch with me.
I felt a great big hollow inside, with a great big gap that could have been filled by another source.
It was not what I wanted.

Yet I was stuck there and needed to find a way forward.

So, I struggled to get back in touch with me, the real me that had somehow got lost,

I lived on anti-depressants for years, with a touch of anti-psychotics, and some calmers from Valium, at least I think that's what it was supposed to do.

I think that a lot of people have lost heart along the way, and not been able to keep up with the bedraggled me.

Only my husband has made that effort day to day, week to week, month to month, and to him I owe my life.

He was always there to support me, and encourage me to get on and move on.

Whereas friends just popped in for a while, and then were gone.

It's easy just to bag and hour of time, and then form a view.

But life is not like that.

Life is a continuum, and that means hour by hour as well as day by day.

So one hour is just like a snapshot, and of course I have had many pictures taken in the past with friends.

What I value most though is the continuous process.

Now my psychiatrist has taken me off the anti-depressants and I only take an anti-psychotic, which seems to be working well.

It keeps my head together, thoughts going forward in one direction, which is indeed a change from the past.

Instead of having that real emptiness to my feelings, I now can feel.

What I feel is that the void in my emotions has gone. I now can feel and I like that.

However, now that I am able to feel I need to be able to feel useful and doing some good.

So, I have been thinking about trying to get a part-time job.

I do voluntary work 2 days a week, at a national HQ of the charity Crimestoppers Trust.

My son asks me each day if I have stopped any crimes.

I like that.

I do fundraising work on the computer, and other tasks, but am not involved in face to face crime, rather the back-up of the support side.

I prefer working behind the scenes, because I find it problematic to be the one up front.

I like to be part of the crew, the team working backstage, rather than the actor on stage.

We all have our preferences, and that is mine.

However, I need to feel useful, and doing voluntary work does not entirely fill that gap.

It provides a base where I can offer my services, for free.

But I need more than that, I would like to have a paid job where people would value my time and me, and I would be financially rewarded for the job I do.

I think this would encourage me to feel that I am making progress and moving forward, and there could be light at the end of the tunnel.

This is what is so depressing for people who are long term ill, that illness becomes a way of life, instead of the gentle progress that we usually find.

So somehow we need to break out of that mould, of depression and emptiness, and join in to the general throng of people who are all making progress together.

Alone we are isolated, but together there is a power, a force, and a synergy.

If I count up the energy I have expended on voluntary work, it is a great deal.

At present I am a school governor, and I also do some work for Merton Volunteer Bureau, visiting isolated housebound older people as well as the charity fundraising.

The local volunteer bureau runs a support group for people with experience of mental health problems, on a Thursday, and I attend these meetings every 2 months.

They are an opportunity t meet up with people who have mental health experience and so there is so much common ground.

We meet with two facilitators, so there is no pressure on the participants who are trying hard to get into their voluntary work and keep a hold on their lives.

Support groups are one way of helping people like us with mental health problems.

Other ways exist.

But more needs to be done.

That is why I am writing these poems and also why I will now write a paper on Developing Structures to help people with mental health problems.

Surely this is the way forward.
We try and help ourselves, but are so dependent on the existing services like the community psychiatrist and medication.
Lord help us and save us from endless medication.
Please show us the way forward.
We need to find a new way ahead.

I Want To Break Free by Anne Brocklesby

I want to break free, I want to be me, again, just me.
I need to be free, to learn to be me.
These words keep going round my head.
They impress themselves upon my mind, just like the music of recover your soul.
When in the grips of mania I think I become quite obsessional and possessive about the words of songs.
It is like a therapy, constant repetition of the phrases that are important to me can really affect me.
I mean they can lift me out of the day to day routine, and into a wider world where I could be free.
John Lennon's Mind Games and Imagine are the same, they move me to feel more of what he was writing about.
I seem to know the meaning of the songs so well, that they drift into my soul.
It is like the meaning of meaning, and the consciousness of the unconsciousness –
We are searching for that inner freedom which we need to really feel.

I think we are searching for God, for an inner peace
which can only come through spirituality.

In my prayer group we learn to pray together in a
shared, secure way.
One person's prayer becomes that of the others, as
we all start to pray together in a spontaneous way.
There is a tremendous power there where we offer
up a prayer to our Lord – Lord hear us.
And the chorus returns with Lord graciously hear
us.
We join our voices and thoughts together around a
theme, which we take as the Gospel of the coming
Sunday.
What does this passage say to us, to you and to me,
it is all valid.
Think awhile and reflect upon the readings and
what others may say.
We gain insight into the teachings of our Lord, and
God's love for us all.
Do not be afraid. Peace be with you.
I am with you even to the end of time.
This is true salvation.
I mean what more could any of us want or need?

Let's Get The Show On The Road by Anne
Brocklesby

Too long we have tarried – I mean how often have
we procrastinated
Or talked so much that we began to suffer from
repeat eardrum syndrome.

There comes a time when you just need to get the show on the road.
I've written about 'Just Convalescing' and 'One Wheel On My Wagon'
Where you feel under par or merely ill-equipped.
But these are the stages that you need to go through to feel ready
It is a process of self-development and management of the self
Where you get to the point of saying one day, well let's get on with it then.
Just do it, is another famous phrase of mine. Yes just do it.

It's time to set the alarm the night before for seven in the morning.
Then chances are that you will want to rise and shine with the bell.
If necessary, buy two more alarm clocks, so that you have three going off
Simultaneously, in different parts of the room.
What a way to get up in the morning.
But it's a way of necessity for so many people.
Those breadwinners who must be at their factory door, or the office desk.
Often long before your alarm has even gone off.
Spare a thought for others in their own showground, so different from yours.

It's the time and the place for action.
We need to be up and doing, aware and being.
Whatever our medium, we need to spread our wings and fly

Higher and higher up above the problems of this sphere
And take an overall perspective.
Like an eagle we need to soar way up above the clouds
Like that clever little wren when we need to be ready to fly
From under the protection of the eagle's wings, when he is tired,
To just peek out above his head and flutter above the rest.

Chapter 33 - Improving Mental Health In The General Population (paper written September 2001)

I am definitely in favour of the appointment of more mental health workers to support those suffering from mental health difficulties in the general population. I see this as beneficial in both the short and the long term, and also very wide reaching. Such a move to provide real practical help for the person who is having mental health difficulties at that time should give a clear insight into the problems faced by the individual and also those within that person's close circle. This would obviously include the 'family', which is reduced to its very basic needs at the time of initial crisis within. For a helper to come in and offer a willing pair of hands, and a listening ear, and practical, quiet support should be a real life-support for the 'victim' of the situation at that point. From this initial immediate crisis input, many changes will arise which should enable real life changes not only for the individual but for the children and the family too.

Crisis intervention is a well known technique for providing assistance when a situation has broken down. Mental health crisis is just such a situation. Existing patterns of behaviour have failed in that situation at that time, and assistance is needed for the change process. A qualified mental health worker, a professional 'in the field' is not used to this kind of 'residential care work'. Such a professional only comes into their own within the emergency situation where an individual is removed to a place of safety, to be cared for elsewhere by other professionals with support staff. Firstly, this kind of approach is false. An individual may manage well, in residential care, away from the pressures which induced the difficulty, but when there is a return, it is to the same situation, although the person themselves may have changed and therefore be unable to cope. Unless of course there is intense work going on within that 'other household' offering complementary/supplementary support to the 'family' or 'carer'. This is really unlikely to be the case ever!

So, we are back at crisis intervention and the provision of extra general support staff within the 'home' setting for the individual who is suffering mental health problems. This focus of 'care' should enable the person to function, at least as well as they were doing prior to the collapse, and also provide some general support in the sense of having a 'buddy' or a 'mentor', a 'pal' or a 'friend'. Of course at the same time, the individual would normally be medically assessed by the GP, the general practitioner, and prescribed medication, or a psychiatrist's appointment, or a community psychiatric nurse, or counselling. Even with the development of new primary care groups and trusts, and the formation of hospital trusts and boards, focus is more defined, but the social model of care is often absent, as the starting point is 'illness' within the medical model. However, new initiatives and cultural developments are emerging. We see outreach work like 'Sure Start' and pilot projects to encourage community participation, including patients, users and carers groups. There are partnership initiatives and protocols. We also see joint training initiatives like shared courses for nurses and social workers establishing the common boundaries and a shared perspective.

But these interventions take time. Emergency psychiatric appointments do not happen immediately, and medication takes time to work, to be adjusted, to accommodate the individual to that stage of the process in which they find themselves. So in the meantime, immediately a helper could be allocated to provide support to a person suffering with mental health difficulties. This at least could be viewed as stabilising the situation, in a sense freezing it in time for that day, that week, that month, and in the course of events, and of a lifetime, that is very little. That point of crisis can be seen as an opportunity for a turning point, a change for the better, with immediate crisis intervention work, followed up by intensive support services as required. This will be the necessary preventative work, and eliminate delayed reactions to stress and loss, perhaps in the next generation, or the one after that. This is the way to break that cycle. Ideally mental health work should also focus in on awareness and prevention, and I do think that message is getting across to certain sections of the population, but there are some to whom the words are completely meaningless. If you are already on the outside, how can you understand what it feels like to be included? Have you ever felt the victim of a conspiracy, or been sent to Coventry? That is temporary. Imagine what it is like to be trapped in an endless tunnel and you cannot see your way out at all.

We need to get a really sound perspective on mental health, which has for too long been regarded as 'their' problem. The long established medical model pronounced by psychiatrists over the centuries is well outdated. A psychiatrist, even a community psychiatrist, is an individual working within his or her professional mode of operation, in the field, and is not there in that person's life at the time. The psychiatrist is a visitor and tries to open windows to perceive and allow perception, but this is not always possible. Especially where the cultural gap is too wide. The window may be newly painted and stuck, or someone may have actually cemented the window in place, to stop the frame from falling out of the wall. Perhaps the window has been barred to prevent criminal access, or the person never wants to open the window for fresh air, because they have become agoraphobic, completely housebound, and at that stage, it is not a psychiatrist, a mind doctor, who is needed, but possibly a psychologist, a behaviour changer, a physiotherapist, possibly a speech therapist, and an aromatherapist to provide that essential complementary care. Again a psychiatric nurse visits and supports at home, but this is intermittent, by nature of appointment, and so is opening a window from within. The next visitor could so easily close that window – perhaps they feel the cold.

Psychiatrists operating within the residential setting are limited as I suggested before, because they are totally removed from the person's own personal life in the community. A psychiatric, psychotherapeutic community is one way to exist, but it is not representative of the full range of life. It is like coasting, where ideas can be explored and huge risks taken without fear of the consequences, but 'life' does not allow that outside. A roller-coaster may give a fun ride, but it comes to an end. We cannot fly like birds, but we could take a flight to another European city, and if the NHS plans for treatment abroad come to fruition, this may soon be available to anyone who needs an operation. Barriers and limitations are always imposed by others who are operating with their own agendas. The sense of self may be very fragile in these circumstances, being buffeted around like an empty wine bottle on the rough seas. A network of mental health support workers available for crisis intervention, support and practical assistance sound the ideal way to keep the person afloat in their own home, which after all is their vessel of choice. The choices may have been very limited, but they are made at a point in time, although constrained by numerous factors.

An increase in mental health support workers in the private homes of individuals will really raise the profile and increase awareness of mental health needs. At present we are just talking about crisis intervention, offering support, but as understanding increases, people will be more prepared to come forward and say could I have a bit of help with a support worker please? We could compare this with the extra support workers who are soon to be available to work in schools. When there are family pressures no one likes to admit they have difficulties, so we struggle on, and life gets into a pattern of coping. Just about coping yes, with this and that, and trouble and loss, and bereavement and separation and extra burdens, and then the finances change and then perhaps you lose the job and then you

start feeling tired and depressed, and then, and then …
It becomes a vicious circle. Mental health problems in
the family affect everyone, and school children need
support with their work at school, in the same way as
employees need family-friendly policies at work.

Looking at the big issue of mental health from another
perspective, the other side of the coin is for those who
have never been loved. For some the pain and the
trouble was always there, but there was no one around
to care, no one who could take on the worries and be
the carer. For some, they have always been the one
who was victimised, always been the one who was not
wanted or not loved enough, or at all, always been the
outsider, who never found anyone to care, or to care
enough. Maybe they just grew tough, said they didn't
care, and found a way of living within that framework.
Maybe they tried to attract our attention, in some way,
by stealing cars, or slitting their wrists, or driving too
fast, or having an accident, or indulging in dangerous
activities, including high risk sport. Maybe, just
maybe, we didn't see, or we didn't understand, but
maybe we were trying hard to get on with our own
difficulties, and maybe no one understood us either.
Maybe we are all in this together, and actually life owes
no one a living, but we need to get on with the talents
we have to make a better world out there. Thinking
about the tortures, atrocities and the despair faced daily
by refugees, homeless, landless, family-less, ward-
driven, and aliens in a strange world which will not
allow them to even come ashore. To promote better
mental health we need to e aware of others' sufferings,
and to work together to change the structures and the

systems which alienate so many of us. A raised awareness of suffering and abuse should bring a greater will into being which wishes to communicate, and to change the perceptions found and sported by many hierarchies of power. When these cultures have been challenged, then we can set to work to build sound structures which an architect would be proud of, and rebuild those strong pillars of wisdom to nurture our children. Mental health difficulties have torn families apart for centuries, and the real innocent victims are the children, trapped in war-torn regions, powerless in the face of the mess which their parents and grandparents have created, No wonder they wish to rebel. Small wonder they do not revolt. There have been stories of American school children, taking arms and returning to the school or college where they grew up, and shooting their teachers and fellow pupils in despair. At other times the focus is on the family, the group of people who have tried their best to make a go of life, to make life work for them – they do not need to be the ones to suffer 'the slings and arrows of outrageous fortune' when one of their members snaps and has no reserves on which to draw. This could be it, for the individual, for the family, for the small groupings of people who have tried to live together and understand each others' problems. However, with support this cold be the turning point for everyone.

The family unit is under increased attack in such a troubled modern city in any part of the world. Pressures to work, to earn enough to support the family, to be a good parent, to give the children a good education, to study hard enough to get a good qualification, at university, college or new opportunities with lifelong learning. No wonder the adult, the parent, or the child collapses. Our inner child says hey, that's enough, I still need to be me, and our own children call out to their parents and say well, where are you, you're mad, what are you all doing out there? We may be adults at 18, but are we really capable of running our own lives and later those of our young dependent children? A balance to life is essential for everyone, but sometimes that is just not there. We all need mental health support workers to say – take a break, cut down that stress, treat yourself now and again, do something for you. We all need people around us who care enough to get involved in our lives and those of our children in our neighbourhood, in our community. We all need support in our lives, in the workplace, in the home, as workers, as parents, as family members. I would see a very busy future for mental health workers in the general population. I do support the government's initiative to provide extra help in the community and the fact that these people have applied to do the job and be paid for it is in one sense a real qualification for the job. They do not come armed with papers which say they are competent to go in and provide caring mental health support, but they show willing to do so, and should be paid appropriately. If you are sitting one day unable to even get up in the morning and it takes at least 2 hours to wash and dress, maybe longer if there are other distractions, like episodes of paralysing fear, or creative imagination takes hold, then how on earth can you cope with a 'life' without a helper. I am totally in support of these extra mental health workers and think they are long overdue.

Post script January 2002: The term 'user' of mental health services is frequently bandied about, but what 'use' does someone have of the professional mental health services? It is a fair question. Rather the 'patient' has to be really patient, and with luck sees the professional service providers on a regular basis, when in 'crisis'. What about the on-going situation – is long-term counselling or practical support offered? Why should there be a cut-off point again? Thinking of the need for help and support, the 'patient/carer/cared for' may require continuing help for a while, or even spasmodically, depending on other factors in their life. We all need to survive, but life is more than survival, where that could be survival of the fittest, as defined in access to resources and care. We could go further and consider the spectrum of continuum of care.

Chapter 34   Post-Script to my Memoirs

I completed my book in October 2003 for the most part, with a few later additions and amendments. One chapter needed to be added, which I have called 'Death In The Family' and is a chapter I wrote after the sudden death of my father, David Blaikie, aged 87 years. His death in December 2003, was totally unexpected, and came as a real jolt out of the blue. To some extent it has kind of rounded off my book, in the sense that my book about manic depression has turned into a book about various forms of grief and early death and how it has affected me. As regards my father, he lived a long and very fulfilled life, and so the grief is tempered with knowledge of a life well lived, with respect and condolences coming from all who knew him. He lived each day and achieved great things in the world of business, serving the community and charity work, and as a grandfather of six young adults, his grandchildren. This time of death was a time of coming together. I met up with my Scottish sister and her two children, and with my other sister and her children whom I see more regularly. Family and friends all congregated together at his funeral service and afterwards at his funeral tea. For the church service, his grandchildren wrote 'A Tribute To A Grandpa', which was read out by my husband. My two children also did readings, including this Gaelic blessing,

"May the roads rise to meet you
may the wind be always at your back,
may the sun shine warm upon your face,

the rains fall soft upon your fields,
and until we meet again,
may God hold you in the hollow of his hand."

To return to my story and subsequent life, I have
continued with my 2 days a week voluntary work with
Crimestoppers Trust and I must say that this has really
been important to me. It has enabled me to get into the
office routine again, and to enjoy coming in to work.
Each and every week over the last year there have been
different tasks for us volunteers to do, and so this has
increased my knowledge of the organisation, and
improved my skills in the various fundraising
techniques. One of my real first successes was the part-
time work the local employment agency asked me to
do. So for a week and a half I actually earned my
living again, working from nine in the morning until
1o'clock doing word processing work for a GP
practice. I really enjoyed getting into the world of
work and felt especially proud when my pay packet
came through at the end of the assignment. I was
appreciated, and the employer had actually paid me to
work. This was a great incentive, and I avidly waited
for more of the same part time work to come my way. I
also started scouring the papers for jobs which appealed
to me. Throughout this time I have continued to attend
the parish prayer group, and as I say, this has always
been there for me – a routine every Thursday afternoon
for myself and all the other regular attendees, and
another lifesaver.

In the meantime, life goes on round about me and I
become involved in various family matters. I'm

finding it a bit easier to take part again, which I see as an important sign of progress.

Through a positive attitude to mental health I am sure we can survive and make more of a contribution to the understanding of mental illness in the community. Let me know what you think.

Write to me at:
Anne Brocklesby
Chipmunkapublishing Ltd
PO Box 6872
Brentwoos
Essex
CM13 1ZT

Chapter 35   A Tribute To My Mother-In-Law

Writing this in February 2007, I have had a quick look over the rest of this book I wrote some years ago. I am surprised at the detail. I also think I must have been inspired to do so much writing and produce the poetry which I enjoy reading now. My mother in law died in December last year, the last of my 3 mothers, and the oldest surviving grandparent to my children. Monica and David together had been a very strong and supportive influence on my development over the years – I knew Monica for 34 years, much longer than my own mother. She helped and supported us and showed us the way ahead – the way forward each day. Monica helped give us the courage to deal with life and the problems it throws at us. Also we know how to enjoy the good times. We have to be the older generation now, there is no one else to rely on. In our fifties we are the ones to whom the younger people look for guidance – it is our job to try not to let people down, so far as we are able.

After a course of CBT – cognitive behavioural therapy – I will soon be embarking upon some psychotherapy. The journey in life continues.

Useful Organisations

Chipmunkapublishing
02075574683
www.chipmunkapublishing.com

MIND
MIND InfoLine 0845 766 0163
www.mind.org.uk

Mental Health Foundation
Telephone: 020 7803 1101
www.mentalhealth.org.uk

The British Association for Counselling and
Psychotherapy (BACP)
Tel: 0870 443 5252
www.bacp.co.uk

The British Psychological Society
Telephone: 0116 254 9568
Produces a directory of chartered psychologists
www.bps.org.uk

Royal College of Psychiatrists
Tel: 020 7235 2351
www.rcpsych.ac.uk

Samaritans
Helpline: 08457 90 90 90 (open 24 hours, seven days a week)
Confidential telephone helpline for anyone who is feeling low, depressed or suicidal. Also offer support in person, by letter or by email.
www.samaritans.org.uk

SANE
Saneline 0845 767 8000
www.sane.org.uk

Printed in the United Kingdom
by Lightning Source UK Ltd.
119557UK00001B/64-81